FROM THE HEART THROUGH THE HANDS

THE POWER OF TOUCH IN CAREGIVING

Dawn Nelson

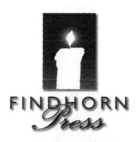

FINDHORN
Press

First published in 2001

ISBN 1-899171-93-2

British Library Cataloguing-in-Publication Data.
A catalogue record for this book is available from the British Library.

Edited by Lynn Barton
Layout by Pam Bochel
Front cover design by Dale Vermeer
Cover photograph by Barry Barankin
Back cover design by Thierry Bogliolo

Printed and bound in the USA

Published by

Findhorn Press

The Park, Findhorn
Forres IV36 3TY
Scotland
Tel 01309 690582
Fax 01309 690036

e-mail: info@findhornpress.com

http://www.findhornpress.com

For Nana

The author and publisher gratefully acknowledge permission from
North Atlantic Books to reprint quotations from
Sunbeams: A Book of Quotations edited by Sy Sanfransky, copyright 1990.

Some passages in this book appeared previously in the work entitled
Compassionate Touch: Hands-On Caregiving for the Elderly, the Ill and the Dying
(Station Hill Press, NY, 1994).

Table of Contents

Preface

This book is for people who like to touch and be touched, and for those who long to be touched more. It is for those who feel comfortable communicating through their hands and for those who wish to feel more at ease in transmitting care through touch. It is for people whose responsibility or job or gift it is to help take care of the elderly and ill members of our society or to oversee that care. It is for sons and daughters caring for aging parents with physical impairments that effect a role reversal in a lifetime of relating. It is for the courageous men and women who continue caring for spouses or mothers or fathers with dementia-related diseases such as Alzheimer's after such a disease has robbed that loved one of the ability to remember the relationship he or she once shared with the caregiver. It is for companions and family members struggling and sometimes sacrificing to provide care for their loved ones at home. It is for the underpaid and overworked C.N.A.'s in skilled nursing communities whose daily duties include providing physical care for men and women experiencing a wide range of physical and mental challenges.

This book is for doctors who have forgotten or never learned that touch is medicine and for those who are wise enough to know that a five-second hug, offered as a gesture of shared humanity, can often do more to assuage fear and anxiety than a five-minute lecture. It is for nurses and nursing assistants who, once trained in giving back rubs to hospitalized patients to reduce discomfort and induce sleep, now may be more often in contact with equipment than with people, forced to spend most of their time dispensing medicines and completing paperwork. It is for the restorative aides, the occupational, physical and recreational therapists, in extended care facilities who are searching for more effective and affirming ways of relating to those whom they serve. It is for compassionate administrators and directors open to implementing cutting-edge modalities and life-enhancing activities for their patients, residents and program participants. It is for hospice professionals and volunteers, hired companions, geriatric consultants, guardians, home health aides and others who want to help improve quality of life for their charges and clients. It is for chaplains and social workers and grief counselors who wish to reclaim the power of intentional touch in ministering to the frail, the distraught and the bereaved. It is for massage therapy students desiring to build careers in arenas that combine service with professional and personal growth and for practitioners whose hearts and hands lead them to forge new paths in venues where their skills are sorely needed. It is for anyone who wishes to use touch more consciously and compassionately in relating to the elderly, the ill and the dying.

ABBREVIATED TITLES USED IN THIS BOOK

A.C.C.	Alzheimer's Care Coordinator
C.M.T.	Certified Massage Therapist
C.N.A.	Certified Nursing Assistant
C.N.S.	Clinical Nurse Specialist
D.O.N.	Director of Nursing
L.C.S.W.	Licensed Clinical Social Worker
L.M.T.	Licensed Massage Therapist
M.A.	Master of Arts
R. N.	Registered Nurse

DEFINITIONS OF TERMS USED

acknowledgment: recognition; a response; confirmation; acceptance

attentive: paying attention; alert, focused, mindful, observant, present

contact: to be in touch with; to make a connection which is not necessarily physical; the flow of energy between two individuals; recognition

individual: something other than the body, mind, emotions or personality; that which is sometimes called true essence, pure being, true nature or other names; that which remains true about another from birth through death regardless of changes in appearance, points of view and so on

intuitive: non-intellectual understanding; direct awareness or knowing; knowledge that is derived from an innate or inner wisdom rather than from logical, linear thinking

skilled: proficient at; competence derived from natural ability or due to specialized training

touch: to place or bring one's hand into physical contact with another; to create a connection with another; to make contact with another; to elicit or evoke a response from another by the quality of attention directed toward him or her

Introduction

As I was emerging from my mother's womb, my father was dodging bullets in the European war zone. My "war bride" mother was young, frightened and ill equipped for single parenting. During my infancy, to assuage her anxieties and loneliness, she began going out in the evenings to have a few drinks in a local bar, leaving me alone after I fell asleep. One fateful night, when I was just over a year old, my mother drank so much that all memory of her parenting responsibilities disappeared in the alcohol-induced fog that infiltrated her mind. I spent the next three days and nights alone—cold, wet, hungry and untouched in my crib. I was ultimately rescued by a neighbor's call to the police about a crying child in a darkened house, transferred to a hospital where I was treated for dehydration and eventually turned over to my fraternal grandparents for custodial care. Like the baby dinosaur "Little Big Foot" in the movie, *Land Before Time* who, when reunited with his grandparents after the big "earthshake" that claimed his mother's life, recognizes them "by their smell, by their love and by their touch," I began to be healed by my grandparents' unconditional love and by their gentle, nurturing touch.

One of my keenest and sweetest early childhood memories is of my grandmother lovingly brushing my hair and "smoothing" my forehead with her fingers as I lay with my head in her lap. My grandfather's hands were firm and reassuring. I can visualize him lifting me up from the ground into the safety of his loving arms, rescuing me from whatever had frightened or upset me until its power has ebbed away. I have a sense memory of my small hand held securely in my grandmother's larger, stronger one as we crossed city streets and walked along sandy beaches looking for shells.

I retain another memory from a time some years later, when I am living with my father and stepmother. My beloved grandparents have finally arrived at our home for a much-anticipated visit while I've shut myself in my room in some adolescent funk or another, hurling myself face down on my bed in a tirade of tears. My grandmother knocks softly at my closed door and slips quietly into the bedroom. Sitting beside me on the bed, her warm hand shapes itself gently around the back of my neck, and then she says something I will never forget. "Do you feel these two little balls in your neck? We get these knots when we're upset or angry but if you rub them and just calm yourself down, they will go away." Without another word, her fingers continue massaging the tense spots in my neck until the bumps do seemingly disappear. Then she holds me, silently, in her arms and lets me cry until my tears cease.

My grandmother not only helped me survive the shock and confusion of my mother's untimely abandonment but continued to touch me and teach me throughout her ninety-three years on earth. She taught me mostly through the constancy of her unconditional love and acceptance.

Another memory of a recurring childhood experience has remained vivid in my body and mind through the years. It has to do with what I was always told were "growing pains." Awakened from sleep by the intensity of aching in my legs, I call out "Daddy, Daddy," until my father rouses himself from slumber and comes to rub my legs. Sometimes we talk and sometimes the ritual plays itself out in silence, yet no matter how many times I call out to him throughout my childhood and adolescence, he appears and he rubs the aching muscles in my legs until I fall back asleep.

I had been a massage therapist for many years when my father was diagnosed with metastasized, inoperable lung cancer. During a weeklong stay in his home a few months before he died, I began giving him foot massages once or twice a day. I did it because it was a skill I possessed, because I wanted so desperately to do something more to relieve his discomfort than hand him pills, and because I longed for any distraction from my grief. He often fell asleep while I was massaging his feet and then I would sit beside him, keeping my attention on him, breathing with him, loving him. Sometimes this exercise helped soften my resistance to his approaching death.

My experience with my father before his death kindled in me a desire to touch others who were in a weakened state, perhaps bedridden and nearing the end of a life cycle. This desire led me to become a hospice volunteer, offering gentle massage and attentive touch to patients and their caregivers. After several months of volunteering, I became a paid member of a hospice caregiving team. During this same period of time, my oldest daughter's staff position in a skilled nursing facility gave me the opportunity to offer age-appropriate massage to a number of older and less mobile adults with a variety of chronic and acute illnesses.

These two venues afforded me a rich education in relating to those in later life stages through touch. One of the first things I learned was that my carefully honed bodywork and massage skills were probably the least important aspect of the work. I learned that appropriate communication skills were essential, patience was primary and remaining open, focused and present was critical. I noticed that a key factor for a successful interaction was the ability to relate to the *individual* regardless of that person's aging process, medical diagnosis, mental state or the condition of his or her physical body.

The response of hospice patients and facility residents to this type of one-on-one attention and nurturing contact was so positive and so gratifying that, at the suggestion of my daughter, I created the COMPASSIONATE TOUCH® Program specifically for the confined elderly and ill in care facility and home settings. I was excited and enthusiastic about making skilled touch available to those who were too old, too weak or too ill to seek out such treatment. I was eager to do something to help enhance the quality of life for those who were isolated, alone, frightened and confused.

The program, which began as a business, evolved eventually into a therapeutic modality which has proven especially effective in palliative care situations for the elderly, the ill and the dying. Before long I began teaching workshops and training others to give COMPASSIONATE TOUCH® sessions. My work continues to be challenging, instructive, satisfying and rewarding in myriad ways. Sometimes it is medicine, meditation and miracle all at once.

After nearly a decade of spending time with countless individuals experiencing AIDS, Alzheimer's, cancer and other debilitating and life-threatening diseases, I unexpectedly became seriously ill myself. Weeks of invasive testing revealed nothing until doctors finally ordered a CT (computerized tomography) scan, which showed that a tumor had grown across my abdomen and into my colon. After a five-and-one-half hour surgery I was diagnosed with a fairly rare and aggressive form of ovarian cancer.

During my hospitalization, treatment and recovery periods, when I was feeling weak, vulnerable, apprehensive, scared and isolated, I experienced quite directly, from my reversed perspective, the profound power of touch in caregiving. The quality of attention and contact I received from those assigned to my care varied vastly. Most of the people who came to my bedside were intent on completing their assigned tasks as quickly as possible. They were dutifully taking care of the patient, yet they failed to see or respond to me! Few called me by name or looked at me directly. When someone did actually contact me and touch me in a gentle, conscious, caring way, it made an enormous difference. Though it did nothing to change the reality of my diagnosis, what the touch accomplished in that moment was to help me feel less alone, less anxious and more whole.

I have come to realize that the pain in my legs was only part of the reason I called out to my father in the middle of the night during my youth. I cried out when I was frightened or lonely or just to see if anyone cared. I wanted reassurance that I wasn't alone. I wanted to make sure someone was there. Because the reassurance my father gave me came in the context of massaging my legs when they hurt, I learned to associate touch with compassion. My grandmother's unconditional regard for me, originally expressed through the intimacy of her tender, hands-on care, created in my mind an inextricable correlation between compassion, touch and love. Some say that compassion is love in action and love—I believe—is the most powerful healer there is.

The Power of Presence

Sandy said that she had become a volunteer in Mother Teresa's ashram in Calcutta because she wanted to understand compassion as something more than an intellectual concept. When she arrived at the ashram, she was given a simple job. Her sole task was to rub oil on the backs of the women who made their way to the ashram—those who were sick in body, in mind or in spirit. In carrying out that duty, Sandy understood "the miracle of touch." One day, a young Indian woman was brought to the ashram after her husband threw hot candle wax over most of her body and put her out into the street. The woman was near death, in great pain, and could not tolerate any physical contact. Sandy realized there was no way to communicate with her verbally since neither woman knew the other's language. Sandy also realized that there was absolutely nothing she could do other than to be there, partnering this woman in the reality of the moment. So she sat down beside her and remained attentive. The two women shared the silence and looked into one another's eyes. Suddenly the Indian woman reached up, pulled Sandy down toward her and kissed her. A few hours later she peacefully died. "And this," Sandy said, "is how I learned about the power of presence."

I find that when massage therapists take my workshops, many of them are expecting me to teach them a series of specific movements or a set of massage techniques which they can then duplicate and use with senior citizens or with a "geriatric" population. I tell participants in my courses that when you're sitting with a ninety-eight-year-old

The most precious gift we can offer others is our presence. Touching deeply is an important practice. We touch with our hands, our eyes, our ears and also with our mindfulness.

THICH NHAT HANH

*We cannot heal others, we can only
heal ourselves so that our presence
will be healing to others.*

IRENE SMITH

*One of my first jobs as a nurse was
with a wealthy, eccentric lady in her
home. This woman, who had
cardiac and psychiatric problems,
had the financial resources to hire a
full-time cook and two full-time
R.N.'s. Touch and music were the
two things that seemed to reach
through her state of being. When
this lady, who had only rare lucid
moments, was agitated, I would just
hold her and sing songs to her. This
was what calmed her. She taught me
how to be present, to experience
what presence is about, and she
helped me tap into my own
creativity.*

MARIAN WILLIAMS, R.N., C.M.T.

woman in a nursing home who is confused, hard of hearing and unable to move her own wheelchair, that woman will not care what massage school you've attended. She will not be interested in knowing whom you've studied with or how many books you've read on the subject of aging. That person only cares that you're willing to sit with her, hold her hand and treat her with the respect and dignity that she deserves. I tell my students that when you have the opportunity to spend some time with a young woman or a middle-aged man dying of AIDS, she or he will not be interested in how many bodywork modalities you've studied or which massage techniques you know. What is important to that person is the fact that you are willing to be there, and that you are willing to touch her or him.

Some people come to my workshops because they have a strong desire to help the suffering. I remind those who train with me, as I remind myself on a regular basis, that on a subtle level, the mental idea or mind state of "helping" sets up an unequal relationship between two people, casting them in roles of strong and weak, capable and incapable, powerful and powerless. In the quest for authentic relationship, it may be necessary to give up our well-intentioned desire to help. This does not mean that we cannot use our skills and abilities to relieve suffering and to offer support to those who need it. It means we must examine our attitudes, our motivations, our attachments to roles and tasks: we must investigate our intention in relationship. We may need to set aside role identifications that create dependent relationships in favor of just opening our hearts, our minds, ourselves, to those whom we wish to serve. If we can commit ourselves to remaining present and in contact with another, whatever unfolds, then the truth of our contact with that other can flow through and between us and the relationship that evolves can instruct and heal both people.

I tell those who are taking my training courses that if you choose to spend a lot of time with those nearing death, in any capacity, you will eventually encounter situations in which nothing you think you know will work and there will be absolutely nothing you can *do*. Such moments offer tremendous potential for growth if we are willing to let go of our attachments to our ideas and images and concepts about looking good, being right and being in control, if we are willing to surrender our techniques, our words, our egos. The finest gift we can give another is our authentic self in the present moment. We can give up "knowing" in favor of simply "being," and we can be present.

Stephen Levine tells a stunning story about a young couple who, after years of saving and planning, arrive at their vacation destination and are soon hiking up a mountain to the beautiful waterfall which they have long yearned to see. As the trail grows steep and narrow, finally they round a corner and the majestic sight is in their view. The sound of the water rushing over the cliffs is deafening. As they pause on the trail to take in the beauty that is at last theirs to behold, the wife steps back to take a picture. A minute or two later, her husband turns around, the joy of the shared moment alive on his face, and his wife is not there. She has disappeared, fallen to her death, her scream no doubt unheard over the roar of the water. All we ever truly have is the present moment. We cannot know when death may unexpectedly intervene in a relationship.

Presence is about "being here now," being accessible, ready, available. Being present means that we are awake, aware, alert. It means that we are able to set aside our preconceptions and prejudices and simply open to the way things are.

The dilemma is that we are all too often so preoccupied with our own concerns, so absorbed in our own inner dialogue, so busy pursuing the future or reminiscing about the past, that we have great difficulty being present. We have trouble being still long enough to be with ourselves, let alone being able to put our unbiased and unconditional attention on another.

It has been said that full living requires full meeting. To be wholly present for another, we must be willing to break out of our isolation and self-fascination. We must endeavor to set aside our love affair with our own thoughts and ignore the myriad distractions that constantly and consistently present themselves. It is our patient, mindful, undiluted presence with others, not our wise advice or counsel, that encourages and allows honest expression and true meetings.

This quality of presence seems to unite all great teachers and healers. There is enormous power in presence. It is the quality that facilitates opening and creates a space for release, for expression, for change and, ultimately, for transformation. When we encounter it, it fulfills our deepest yearnings and satisfies our deepest needs. Presence predicts and promotes healing, in its deepest sense, because it dissolves separation, restoring the relationship that allows us to experience our wholeness.

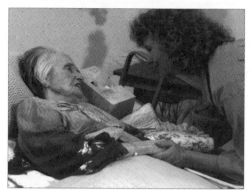

Photographer: Owen Howson

The Compassionate Touch

I listened as the woman sitting across from me spoke about how much she loved her husband and what a kind and decent man he was—a thoughtful lover, a good provider, a loving father to their two young children. She recalled the warm summer evening when he offered to walk to the corner grocery to pick up an item or two to complete their evening meal. In my mind's eye I could see her and her two young daughters setting the table and preparing the rest of the food in anticipation of his return. I could see her moving across the kitchen to pick up the telephone when it rang.

My partner in the class exercise stopped speaking for a moment as tears welled in her eyes and began to roll down her face. Her voice deepened and hardened as she recited the never to be forgotten words spoken in her ear by the voice on the other end of the line. I began to steel myself against what I sensed was surely coming. I didn't want to hear the rest of the story.

When she arrived at the hospital, her husband's body was unrecognizable. A speeding truck careening around the corner felled him just as he stepped off the curb—grocery bag in his arms—to cross the street that would have brought him home. He died in the emergency room without ever regaining consciousness. As my classmate re-lived those moments that so dramatically changed her life, I realized that her words were reaching my ears, yet I was not letting them into my heart. I didn't want to experience her pain or to accept the possibility that such a thing could happen to me. In the same moment I realized that unless I was willing to accept the

I believe that at every level of society—familial, tribal, national and international—the key to a happier and more successful world—at every level of society—is the growth of compassion.

THE DALAI LAMA

Our task must be to free ourselves... by widening our circles of compassion to embrace all living creatures...

ALBERT EINSTEIN

As a mother at risk of her life watches over her only child, so let everyone cultivate a boundlessly compassionate mind toward all beings.

THE BUDDHA

Compassion simply stated is leaving other people alone... You are available to another human being, to provide what they need, to the extent that they ask.

RAM DASS

While I was volunteering for an organization called, "Friendly Visitors," I went to an eighty-one-year-old lady's house to help her with housekeeping. She was very quiet, just sitting at the kitchen table while I worked and made small talk... As I was getting ready to go I asked if she wanted me to blow out the candle. She just kept looking at the candle burning, in broad daylight, and said, "No it keeps me company." I was stopped in my tracks. I didn't know what to say, how to respond or what to do. I sat down and as she looked at me I saw the depth of loneliness. Tears welled up. Sitting quietly with her, silently crying, sharing her desolation and the possibility of mine, brought us together for a brief moment in time.

SANDRA BURNS, L.M.T.

possibility of my own suffering, I could not be truly present to receive hers. I made a decision to open to this woman's sorrow. As I did so, my own tears began to flow and my heart began to ache. There was absolutely nothing I could do or say to change the fact of her loss. As I received her grief, it was as if my mind visited her heart for an instant. I felt the tiniest spark of what she felt and that moment gave birth to my compassion.

Compassion ignites the impulse to relieve the suffering of another. Perhaps inherent in such a response is the ability to set aside our own concerns for a time in order to notice someone else's discomfort, sorrow or need for contact, to let go of preoccupations with our own needs in order to focus on someone else's predicament.

The compassionate heart is affected by the suffering of another. As the heart opens, so do the hands; and the impulse to reach out and touch the one who is suffering naturally follows. Compassion supports an ability to offer help appropriate to the need. It may direct the desire to assist another in some way such as driving that person to the grocery store, cooking a meal, painting a house or giving money or material goods that help ease some hardship. It may generate an offer of hands-on support such as dressing a wound, lotioning a body or giving a back rub. Sometimes, compassion simply activates our attention. It urges us to awaken, to see more fully, to listen more carefully. It allows us to see and to hear not just with our eyes and our ears, but with our hearts. Compassion is what allows us to accept the reality of a difficult situation and to remain consciously present, for even a few moments, in that reality with another human being.

Compassion implies an experience of unconditional regard for an individual irrespective of that person's gender, race, culture, physical appearance, belief system, disease process or mental capacity. It implies a genuine, sincere interest in that person's well-being and it supports an ability to offer whatever aid is needed.

For humankind to thrive and evolve, it is essential that we find ways to nurture and express our compassion. When we make the effort to discard our exclusive preferences, detach from our points of view, our belief systems and our opinions, simply opening our hearts to our fellow human beings, whatever the condition or circumstance, we clear a space for compassion to grow.

I believe that touch is a basic human need, essential to our survival, and that the therapeutic benefits of touch for both the giver and the receiver are undervalued. There is a subtle but significant difference between conscious physical contact and casual, random touch. Intentional touch as an expression of compassion and as an aid in healing has a long history. The therapeutic use of hands is an ancient example of the ability of humans to serve one another through touch and appears to be a universal healing act.

References to rubbing and to anointing with oil, as well as terms such as friction, squeezing, vibration, pressure, percussion and stroking, have evolved into to the more general word, *massage* (probably from the Arabic meaning "to touch or to handle"), which is used today to refer to a broad range of touch and bodywork modalities. Our ancestors discovered the connection between physical touch and well being long before science felt the need to prove that such a relationship exists. Evidence of the use of massage "is demonstrated in ancient traditions which continue to be handed down from teacher to pupil in India, Tibet, and China; in the early rock carvings of Egypt and Chaldea… and in the accounts of certain historical figures."[1]

The Greeks and Romans, famous for their baths, spas and temples of healing, believed that massage could aid in relief of pain as well as in developing strong and healthy bodies. Touch was an integral part of Jesus' healing ministry as an expression of his compassion; and the lying on of hands was used extensively by his early followers. A Hindu sculpture of a reclining god, Vishnu, at the National Museum in Bangkok, Thailand shows two celestial helpers massaging his legs.[2]

Massage in a variety of forms has been a key element in Ayuvedia, practiced in India for 5,000 years and has long been an integral part of traditional Chinese medicine. Native American tribal healers have traditionally cared for the infirm and the elderly by rubbing their bodies with oils and spices; and early European physicians routinely prescribed massage as a pain-relieving remedy.

Happily, massage as a healing modality is re-emerging in present day healthcare, once again gaining recognition, not just as a indulgence for the rich and the pampered but as a respected and credible form of therapy and even a basic part of wellness care.

Touch that is healing and nourishing can be administered by anyone who feels inspired to reach out toward a fellow human being. Indeed, the impetus to share our energy in this particular way often arises spontaneously and intuitively when our hearts open to those around us who are in need of contact, encouragement and support.

We have to find ways to nourish and express our compassion.

THICH NHAT HANH

Our instinctive reaction to injury is to touch the painful area or the person who is hurt. When we experience discomfort, our hands automatically go to the point of pain. Even when our hurts are internal, we use touch to comfort ourselves and offer solace to others through strokes and hugs and tender pats. Parents of almost every race and culture touch their babies and children to soothe them when they are upset, and to nurse them when they are hurt, as a symbol of love. Anyone can cultivate and nurture the natural compassion of the heart.

The compassionate touch emanates not from the hands but from the heart. Our natural impulse to comfort both others and ourselves through touch activates the heart/hand connection. In following that spark, we ignite the flame of compassion in our hearts, allowing it to warm, inform and flow through our hands. In reaching out to another, the touch that originates in the heart of the giver has the potential to connect with more than the physical form of the receiver. It has the power to connect two souls in a mutual recognition of their shared humanity and their yearning to be healed.

A Word to Nonprofessional and Professional Touch Practitioners

Some people are hesitant to use touch techniques in caregiving because they think they cannot do so without formalized training. It is true that in most areas, you cannot and should not charge money for massage services or advertise yourself as a massage practitioner unless you have completed a course of training from an accredited school that allows you to become certified or licensed to do so. However, unless you want to pursue a professional career in massage, it is not necessary to go through what can be an expensive and exhaustive formalized training program. Almost anyone who desires to do so can increase his or her knowledge and skill in administering touch and can develop the ability to utilize touch as a resource in caregiving.

Many people have an innate, natural ability to use their hands to soothe and satisfy others. I have encountered many men and women who have never formally studied massage or bodywork techniques who, nonetheless, instinctively know how to touch someone in a comforting and healing way. Many parents administer touch therapy regularly to their children without even thinking about it. The ability to know when, where and how to calm their child through touch grows out of their love.

In the weeks leading up to her death, I sometimes gave my mom foot rubs, which she loved. Her skin was drying and I would stand at the end of her bed massaging her feet with skin cream. I've never been trained in massage, but I think it is a natural art. When hands hold feet, and there is a loving relationship there, a natural massaging action begins to take place. No training seems to be required. I experienced the same phenomenon while holding her hands. These massages gave Mom a special kind of relief. She would sigh, as if surprised that her body was still capable of feeling good sensations. These times were a special form of communion between us.

LAWRENCE NOYES

Touch is at the heart of everything.

ZACH THOMAS, *HEALING TOUCH:
THE CHURCH'S FORGOTTEN
LANGUAGE*

In the context of touch in palliative care, I believe there are several talents more significant than the knowledge of specific massage techniques. One is the ability to truly put your attention on the individual whose body you are touching. If you are able to "see" an individual, as opposed to simply looking at a body, and you are able to reach out to that individual with a caring and open heart, your touch is likely to be far more effective than that of a highly trained professional who may be simply going through the mechanics of manipulating a physical body. Assuming you feel comfortable and at ease communicating through touch; and if you are in contact with the individual, I believe that you will intuitively know what to do and how to proceed in making a physical connection. Your heart will guide your hands.

If you are a volunteer or family caregiver and you want to increase your ability to use touch more skillfully, you can learn some basic and simple techniques by taking a class or weekend workshop from an experienced and reputable teacher, and even from reading books on the subject. There are several good books on the market that include pictures, drawings and clear instructions on how to practice basic massage techniques. Practice on healthy people first, offer to trade short massage sessions with a family member, friend or colleague and then give each other feedback, making sure to emphasize what was positive or effective about the other person's touch. Direct experience is always the best teacher! Another thing you can do is get massage or bodywork sessions yourself from an experienced practitioner. Notice what relaxes you and notice what qualities the practitioner has (or does not have) that make you feel at ease (or not).

Most of the touch, relaxation and communication techniques detailed in this book can be utilized by both professional and nonprofessional healthcare providers and volunteer or family caregivers. Many of them can be integrated into daily caregiver tasks, offered during routine visits or used during a special period of time set aside for a touch session.

If you have studied a particular form of massage or bodywork modality, and are an experienced professional practitioner, you will need to assess your comfort level in being with elderly and ill people and in the healthcare setting. If your feel at ease in such settings, then you need only adapt your skills to working with these special populations, and perhaps get some additional specialized training to build your confidence and expand your knowledge.

Accessing the bodies of people confined to beds or wheelchairs who are experiencing a variety of physical and mental challenges is quite different from working with younger, healthier people on a massage table. Techniques that might be used in doing therapeutic massage or bodywork in a spa or sports setting, for instance, are not always possible, appropriate or desirable when massaging the bodies of the aged, the ill and those nearing death.

There are other differences as well. In a private massage practice, you create an environment conducive to relaxation in the room in which your massage table is set up. You control everything from the height of the table to the color of the walls in the room. You can change the placement of the massage table and other articles in the room; you can adjust the temperature of the room or warm the table with a heating pad. You can vary the scents and the sounds in the room to address individual preferences. You can hang plants, light candles, place flowers and dim the lights or draw the curtains to create a more peaceful atmosphere.

Offering massage or touch therapy sessions to people in care facilities or in their own home environments means that you must adapt to a variety of spaces which are often quite the opposite of what you might prefer. The atmosphere may be anything but restful. Space is often limited and there are few options for making any changes. There are likely to be many distractions and distinctive sounds and smells, over which you have no control.

Your client may reside in a room with two or three other people. The person in the next bed may be watching television or conversing with visitors. There is no way to block out sounds or to insure privacy other than a cotton cloth hanging between the two beds. Space may be limited. Interruptions during touch sessions are not uncommon.

The length of the massage session is another difference to consider. An active healthy person can usually tolerate one hour or longer of deep massage and/or full-body work. A touch session with a frail elderly or seriously ill person may be only fifteen to twenty minutes in duration. In general, any massage techniques used during such a session should be softer, gentler and practiced for a shorter period of time than those which are used in other kinds of therapeutic massage and bodywork sessions.

There are people for whom the word "massage" has negative connotations. It may conjure up visions of a body being kneaded into a bruised pulp or it may be linked with something of an illicit or sexual nature. A friend and colleague of mine began a career as a touch therapist, in her seventh decade of life, as a volunteer at a Veterans Administration Hospice Unit. She got a lot of negatives responses when she asked patients if they wanted a massage but soon learned that if she offered a back rub there were lots of eager takers.

Even though I often do use certain kinds of massage techniques in working with the elderly and the ill, I seldom use the word massage in introducing myself to someone. If the person is verbal and conversant, I sit down and establish some rapport with the person first. Then, I usually ask if he or she would like a back rub or like some hand lotion applied. If the word "massage" does come up, I let the person know that he or she does not have to get out of bed, go anywhere else or remove any clothing.

At some point during the visit I might put some lotion on my hands and then ask the person if she'd like some on her hands also. If a person is hesitant about being touched, I might bring out a finger puppet or other object to engage the person in a tactile experience that is less threatening than direct physical contact. I also let the person know that we can just sit and visit. I never insist on touching someone or try to talk anyone into any kind of massage or physical contact if he or she, at that moment, is not open to being touched.

Her touch was so gentle and it warmed my hands and I felt wonderful after her visit!

EVA BRAND,
RETIREMENT HOME RESIDENT

Professional Massage Organizations:

American Massage Therapy Association
    820 Davis Street, Ste.100, Evanston, Illinois 60201
    Phone: 847-864-0123
    Fax: 847-864-1178
    email: info@inet.amtamassage.org
    Web-site: www.amtamassage.org

Associated Bodywork & Massage Professionals
    28677 Buffalo Park Road, Evergreen, CO 80439
    Phone: 1-800-458-2267
    email: expectmore@abmp.com
    Web-site: www.abmp.com

Hospital-Based Massage Network
    612 S. College Avenue, Ste. 1, Ft. Collins, CO 80524
    Phone: 970-407-9232
    Fax: 970-225-9217
    Web-site: www.HBMN.com

National Assoc. of Nurse Massage Therapists
    P.O. Box 820, Clarksdale, AZ 86324
    Phone: 1- 800-262-4017
    email: simpson@sedona.net
    Web-site: www.members.aol.com/nanmtl

Volunteer Organizations:

There are a number of hospice and other volunteer organizations that include touch training or a touch component in their programs or that would welcome massage therapists on their volunteer rosters. Contact:

    National Hospice Organization
    1901 N. Moore Drive, Suite 901, Arlington, VA 22209
    Phone 703-684-7722

Some volunteer organizations exist for the sole purpose of providing touch and related services to the ill and the elderly who are homebound or hospitalized. One such organization is:

    The Heart Touch Project
    1025 Indiana Avenue, Venice, CA 90291
    Phone 310-451-6112
    Fax 310-452-6272
    email: mailhearttouch@aol.com
    Web-site: infor@hearttouch.org

The Efficacy
of Touch

Modern medical technology offers many life-saving and life-prolonging procedures, yet it often fails to treat the whole person. Health care has become equated with costly procedures and, according to one professor of nursing, "thousands of people visit physicians' offices every year just to be touched."[3] With the great variety of advanced medical techniques and pain-relieving drugs available in today's world, one basic and fundamental element of healing has been all but forgotten—the simple, care-full touch of the human hand. Although touch is one of oldest and most effective means available for relieving discomfort in the body, reducing stress and inducing a state of relaxation, it is only beginning to be rediscovered in the healthcare community.

Recent research indicates that massage can boost the immune system by increasing lymphatic flow, one of the body's primary defenses against infection. This discovery has far-reaching implications in the search for ways to ward off opportunistic infections in those with compromised immune systems. It is now thought that massage may stimulate the release of endorphins, the body's natural painkillers, into the brain and nervous system. The physiological reaction to caring touch, it is currently postulated, helps rebalance the flow of nerve chemicals within the brain, called neurotransmitters, which may be responsible for the feelings of well-being or euphoria that often follow a massage or touch session.[4]

Administered consciously and skillfully, touch has enormous power to ease discomfort, relax the body, calm the mind and lift the spirit. It

The prevalence of pain in elders is known to be twice that of younger individuals; in community-residing elders, the prevalence of pain ranges from 25 percent to 50 percent. In long-term care settings, the prevalence of pain can be as high as 85 percent.

PAIN MANAGEMENT PROTOCOL,
GERIATRIC NURSING, SEPT.–OCT., 1996

I offer geriatric massage in fifteen-minute sessions at a care facility. A family member stopped me in the hall and asked if I could come in and do a session with her mom who had suffered a stroke and had hemiperises on her right side. The daughter had been trying to get her mom's right hand to open up with no success. I worked on all the muscles in the contracted hand for fifteen minutes, and it opened up. The daughter was totally amazed!

JANET McPHERSON, R.N., L.M.T.

offers reassurance and support to those who are anxious and troubled. It helps restore a sense of worth and value to those who are frail of body and mind.

It nurtures and nourishes those who are starved for human affection and contact.

Among the aged, in particular, the course, as well as the duration, of many minor illnesses can be greatly influenced by the quality of physical contact and tactile support that an individual receives. The right touch, given at just the right moment, can, in and of itself, be immensely healing. I do not mean healing in the sense of reversing the aging process or of taking away a disease or a disability—but healing that equates with the root meaning of the word *health*, which is "wholeness"—healing that allows awareness to expand beyond physical or mental discomfort to a larger reality of completeness and well-being.

PHYSICAL BENEFITS

The losses and infirmities that frequently accompany advancing age and illness carry with them the potential for long-term stress. Massage has a proven history of efficacy as a primary or adjunct therapy for almost any condition that includes a stress component. As tension and stress are relieved, minor physical ailments sometimes disappear. A reduction in bodily tension promotes an overall relaxation response, which, in turn, can produce benefits such as

- greater ease in breathing
- increased mobility
- increase in appetite
- improved digestion and elimination

Eliciting a relaxation response contributes to a lessening of anxiety, which can effectively soothe the body, quiet the mind and strengthen the spirit. The vicissitudes of aging may seem less overwhelming. In other words, the relaxation response can cause a chain reaction of positive benefits within the body/mind.

Gentle touch and sensitive, age-appropriate massage, whether administered by a professional practitioner, a caring volunteer, a life-long companion or a knowledgeable friend, can help reduce the general level of nervous tension in the body. This release in muscular tension can

- decrease the need for pain medication
- result in more restful sleep
- help increase mobility
- improve balance and coordination

Poor circulation is a major concern for the bedridden ill and for those who become less and less mobile due to the frailties of aging. In simplified terms, adequate circulation of blood and lymphatic fluids in our bodies is normally accomplished by the constant contraction of muscles pressing against our veins and capillaries as we move about in daily activities. Injury, illness or inactivity inhibits these natural processes, and decreases circulation in the body. Although exercise is the best and quickest way to increase circulation, it is not always possible. Regular massage can assist the flow of blood and encourage lymphatic flow. Improving circulation in the body can help

- prevent or reduce edema
- prevent pressure sores
- speed healing from surgical procedures
- increase energy
- improve skin tone and color
- promote better sleep

Whether it is given in the form of a gentle back rub, a foot massage or simply focused physical contact, touch is beneficial to the elderly in multiple and synchronous ways.

As the aging process continues, elders frequently become less and less active. A variety of physical impairments and challenges often contributes to decreasing mobility. Long-term immobility is a major factor in poor circulation; and poor circulation can lead to other symptoms such as

- inertia
- shortness of breath
- loss of appetite
- mental confusion
- depression

Even very gentle therapeutic massage techniques help stimulate the nervous system and increase the oxygen-carrying capacity of the blood throughout the body. People are sometimes able to rest more easily or sleep less fitfully after a massage or touch session. Some experience increased mental clarity; some report feeling less despondent or more "alive."

Hospital patients are encouraged to get up and walk as soon as possible after surgical procedures because any form of movement will increase circulation, and increased circulation speeds healing and recovery. Touch techniques that help promote better circulation in the body also contribute to rebuilding of tissue and thus help speed the healing process.

Insomnia can be caused from any number of physical and emotional distresses as well as from environmental conditions. An ill or aged person's inability to sleep well can become an additional source of stress for that that person as well as for his or her caregivers. Focused, caring touch has a tranquilizing effect on many people. As the body relaxes and tension decreases, a person may be able to breathe more easily and more deeply. Greater ease in breathing can facilitate more tranquil and restful sleep. It is not uncommon for people to doze off during a touch session. Regular touch sessions can reduce the need for sleep-inducing medications.

There are many reasons for loss of appetite among the aged. Those living alone, with no one else to cook for or to share food with may slowly loose interest in preparing and eating food. Those with memory loss may literally forget when to eat or if they have eaten. Drug and chemotherapy treatments, constipation, nausea and vomiting, pain, weakness and fatigue, mouth problems, liver and pancreatic disorders can all affect the appetite. Anxiety and general malaise or depression can affect one's desire to eat. One-on-one

21

Let us be kinder to one another.
ALDOUS HUXLEY'S LAST WORDS

I had the privilege of working with F. and her family off and on for nearly two years. She had a rare form of cancer that had settled in her spine. The tumor was actually wrapped around her spinal cord so that it could not be completely removed surgically without severing the cord. The cancer was discovered during a battery of tests conducted after F. fell down one day as she was crossing a busy street. At the time I met her, F. was not only bedridden but, due to an increasing paralysis in her legs, was practically immobilized. She could turn her neck and shoulders but could not turn her body on her own. Pressure sores were a constant problem for her. She once remarked that they happened so quickly and yet seemed to take forever to heal. Regular massage helped to speed the healing of several fairly severe pressure sores and to prevent additional skin breakdown and discomfort.

AUTHOR

attention, along with a reduction in stress and better circulation in the body, can promote better digestion as well as increase the desire for food and drink.

Constipation is a common problem among the aging and is a side effect of many medications prescribed for a variety of ills. Constipation may also be due to inactivity and lower fluid intake. It is a problem that can be extremely irritating, frustrating and uncomfortable. Constipation is usually treated through diet and mild laxatives. Gentle abdominal massage can be helpful in stimulating bowel activity. Reducing a person's general stress level and increasing circulation in the body can also help ease elimination problems.

Loss of skin elasticity and dryness are natural effects of the aging process in the body. Dehydration, immobility, using multiple medications and a generally rundown condition can also contribute to skin degeneration. Moisturizing the skin frequently becomes more important as aging continues, as does the need for tactile stimulation.

One of the most persistent problems of confinement and decreased mobility among the elderly and the ill is susceptibility to pressure sores (also called bedsores, pressure ulcers or decubitus ulcers). Pressure sores can be a serious threat to health and comfort. These painful ulcerations occur when a prominent part of the body, such as the spine, is pressed continuously against a relatively hard surface such as a mattress or chair so that nutrients and oxygen are prevented from reaching the skin cells of that particular area. Parts of the body especially prone to pressure sores include

- the sacrum, or base of the spine
- shoulders
- elbows
- buttocks
- heels
- ankles

Factors in risk assessment for pressure sores include

- general state of health
- skin integrity
- fluid intake
- types of medication being taken

At highest risk for pressure sores are those who are

- bedridden
- confined to a wheelchair
- no longer able to control bladder or bowel functions
- confused or sedated
- paralyzed
- immobile

The first sign of a pressure ulcer is redness on the skin. If this reddened area is not tended to, the skin can deteriorate until it becomes an open wound. In extreme cases, the deterioration can become so severe that muscle and bone are exposed.

One of the main reasons that nurses and other caregivers are instructed to turn patients who are unable to turn themselves every few hours is to guard against pressure sores. People who sit in wheelchairs for most of their waking hours are encouraged to shift their position every fifteen minutes. However, many wheelchair-bound people are forgetful, and staff members may not have, or may not take, the time to remind or assist them to change positions as frequently as necessary.

Nursing manuals have always included massage instruction in sections on how to deal with this very real and challenging aspect of caring for the less mobile elderly and ill. Lotioning and gently massaging areas of the body that have been most recently under pressure helps stimulate circulation in those areas and is one of the best ways to prevent pressure sores.

Urine or feces left in contact with the skin can also cause skin deterioration fairly quickly, which is why maintaining good hygiene and keeping the skin of those who are bedridden clean and dry is so important. Objects pressed against the skin over a long period of time, such as a watch, a wrist restraint or even a tube connection, can also cause redness and irritation. Shifting the position of the object and renewing the circulation in that area, using lotioning and gentle massage, can easily alleviate this discomfort.

Itching is another fairly common complaint among the bedridden elderly. The cause of the itching can be traced to a variety of causes and sometimes a little detective work is called for. Some types of rashes, skin breakdown, allergic reactions to a particular medication or even laundry soap can cause itching. Moisturizing and massaging the skin may help alleviate this annoying symptom. If the condition persists a medicated or topical cream may be needed and healthcare professionals should be alerted.

Touching or massaging over an itching or weeping rash that could be contagious or that might be spread to other parts of the body should, of course, be avoided. When in doubt about whether a skin condition is contagious, find out before touching or massaging directly on the area.

Psoriasis is one inflammatory skin disease that can look quite alarming in its acute state. It is characterized by reddish patches and white scales and can cause itching. Psoriasis, however, is not contagious, and gentle massage over such a condition can be extremely soothing to the sufferer.

It is good for the skin be kept clean and dry. Sweating is a fairly common problem for the ill. It can occur for no apparent reason, or it may be caused by anxiety, reaction to medication, sudden changes in body metabolism or by fever. A little powder sprinkled and lightly massaged into the skin in areas of the body susceptible to sweat, such as under arms or large breasts, can help with this problem.

Most seriously or chronically ill patients experience some degree of physical discomfort during the course of their disease process and treatment. The pain can be severe, chronic and debilitating. Anxiety and anger, as well as depression, can intensify the perception of pain. Drug therapy is the major modality used for relieving and managing pain; yet drug therapy alone is not always effective, and all drugs have side effects. In more enlightened medical communities, massage is now considered an effective adjunctive (used in addition to or along with a primary treatment) measure for pain control in palliative care.

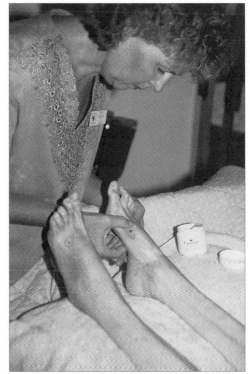

Photographer: Barry Barankin

One of the participants in my workshop that weekend, an experienced physical therapist, encountered a man in a wheelchair sitting by the elevator. His pant legs were rolled up to above his knees revealing a severe case of psoriasis nearly covering both of his exposed limbs. She explained why she was in the facility that day and asked if he might like a back massage which he was quite agreeable to. After a brief back massage, this intuitive workshop participant deftly moved to the gentleman's legs and began gently touching the reddened and swollen skin. Tears began to roll down his face until he was nearly overcome with emotion. His gratitude for her wise and compassionate touch and attention was immense.

AUTHOR

I feel so alive when someone touches me.

PSYCHOSOCIAL BENEFITS

A decade ago, a federal panel assigned by the U.S. government to study ways to improve medical care and lower costs urged greater use of drug alternatives such as massage and relaxation techniques in their guidelines. Such techniques are beginning to be recognized for their usefulness in pain management and in reducing the need for potent and expensive drugs which often have serious side effects requiring treatment with more drugs!

The need to be touched does not disappear with childhood. The benefits of touch hold true through all stages of life and certainly do not diminish in aging. A few medical schools, including Harvard and Duke, are beginning to provide specialized instruction in touch and massage for physicians-in-training. We may hope that touch as a healing art will once again become an accepted part of the physicians bedside manner, and massage as medicine will be considered as part of treatment programs for people of all ages.

Massage is also helpful in reducing tension and muscle spasms that are the result of injury or of years of stored up and repressed emotions. The sedative effects of massage cause a reflex reaction of the nerves that decreases muscle tension. This sedative effect on the nerves may also account for the decrease in pain impulses carried by the nerves to the brain.

Stress is defined as an automatic physical and physiological reaction experienced as the bodily tension we feel when faced with a situation that is new, unpleasant or threatening. Change is known to be a major cause of stress. This fact makes the elderly especially prone to stress since the very fact of aging can include major, multiple and irreversible life changes such as

- retirement
- chronic or acute illness
- death of life companion which may lead to
  - living alone for first time
  - no one to "take care of" for first time
  - change in income or financial anxiety
- illness and/or death of long-time friends
- changes in functional abilities leading to loss of independence such as
  - no longer being able to drive
  - no longer being able to participate in favorite sports or activities
  - becoming less mobile
  - change in residence resulting in
    - moving from large family home to smaller or shared space
    - moving from independent living to assisted living
    - decrease in personal space, personal belongings and privacy
    - loss of familiar surroundings, neighbors, friends and community
    - change in lifestyle and familiar activities

Stress affects the body causing muscular tension and tightness. Other physical signs of stress can include

- headache
- cold hands and feet
- stiff neck
- perspiration
- backache
- constipation or diarrhea
- fatigue
- changes in sleeping and/or eating habits
- insomnia
- shortness of breath

Stress affects the emotions causing worry and anxiety and contributing to emotional feelings and mental states such as

- helplessness
- confusion
- frustration
- sadness
- irritability
- depression
- anger
- inertia
- vulnerability

While a certain amount of stress can be positive, too much stress or prolonged stress can be unpleasant and unhealthy. Stress can exacerbate almost any chronic physical weakness or condition. Stress is thought to be a major factor in causing hypertension, coronary heart disease, migraine and tension headaches, ulcers and asthmatic conditions and is suspected to aggravate chronic backache, arthritis, allergies, vertigo, MS and hyperthyroidism.[5] Stress is also associated with gastrointestinal disorders such as colitis and gastritis. Dermatologists have found stress to be a factor in many skin diseases such as hives, eczema and dermatitis. Some of the excess hormones released by the adrenal glands during repeated stress responses can lower the body's immunity making the person under stress more susceptible to bacterial infections and viruses such as flu.[6]

The effects of stress are cumulative. In other words, a string of small upsets, or constant little stresses, can add up and eventually produce greater health problems.

For the elderly, especially those who live alone or reside in care facilities, loneliness, isolation, multiple and continual losses and fear of abandonment can also become significant sources of anxiety and stress, as can the aging process itself. Long-term stress can lead to depression and can exacerbate feelings of hopelessness and helplessness.

Stress affects the way people feel and think. A person who becomes irritable and irrational from continued high-level stress often passes his or her irritability on to others, creating a kind of ripple effect in relating.

All of us benefit from touch. You can be quite isolated without touch and very lonely... there's something about that skin to skin touch and having another human being caring and touching you that makes you feel good about yourself on the inside.

EVELYN YOUNGBERG, D.O.N.

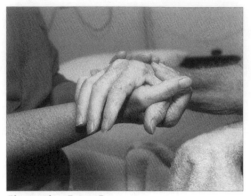

Photographer: Bonnie Burt

I remember sitting with a woman who had been in a coma for several months. I kept my attention on her for awhile and then began lotioning her arms with slow, stroking movements. I was massaging one of her hands when she suddenly took a deep breath followed by a long exhalation and sigh. It could have been coincidence, but I believe it was most likely a response to the human contact and touch she was receiving.

AUTHOR

Muscles contract under stress! When a muscle remains tense over a period of time, actual soreness in the muscle can result due to a buildup of lactic acid in the tissue. One does not have to be an athlete or a construction worker to develop sore muscles. Muscles can become tight and knotted from anxiety, fear, held- in sadness or anger and even from thinking negative thoughts. A pattern emerges in which stress produces tension and discomfort. That discomfort, in turn, produces more stress.

Age-appropriate massage and simple focused, attentive touch techniques can help significantly in stress reduction and stress management for the elderly and the ill. Regular gentle touch massage sessions can be quite effective in helping reduce muscular tension. As muscular tension disappears, anxiety is lessened, triggering a relaxation response and thus reducing overall stress tendencies. As tight muscles soften, tensions ease, the mind and heart open, and the person being touched may relax on deeper levels and begin to experience a sense of calmness and tranquility.

It has been observed in intensive care units that patients in a coma often appear to be more at peace after they are touched. Such patients register improved heart rate and brain waves when their hands are held, even if it is only for the purpose of checking a pulse. Men and women whose bodies are partially paralyzed or who are unable to speak, as the result of a stroke, for instance, often respond to touch in subtle but noticeable ways. Occasionally there is little visible movement or discernable recognition from the person being touched, yet frequently there are observable responses such as

- eyes opening, shutting or blinking
- the jaw relaxing or dropping open
- a sounded sigh
- tears welling in eyes
- a change in the breathing pattern
- head turning
- eye contact
- closed fist opening

Touch as a therapeutic modality can be a significant factor in treating despondency in the aging and the ill because it has the potential to produce multiple psychosocial, mental, emotional and physical benefits. Anyone who works in a retirement, convalescent or nursing facility will tell you that depression can become a major problem among residents. The malaise in some care centers is almost palpable.

The less active elderly and the chronically ill are prone to periods of depression for a variety of reasons both physical and emotional. As the aging process continues and/or an illness progresses, there may be ongoing and increasing physical discomfort. As already mentioned, loss and change are considered major components in stress; and prolonged stress can lead to depression. Change becomes inevitable and can include loss of mental and physical abilities, career, financial security, home, loved ones, and eventually perhaps even bodily functions. The biggest loss may be loss of independence and control over one's life. Mental anxiety and fear—of increased pain, further loss, physical impairment, injury, incapacitation and dying also contribute to depression among the aged. Boredom, loneliness, isolation, feelings of becoming less and less "attractive" or more and more "useless" may contribute to melancholia and erode feelings of self-esteem and self-worth.

Ashley Montagu says that the use of touch and physical closeness may be the most important way to communicate to ill and aged persons that they are still important as human beings.[7] Touch deprivation is a largely ignored yet major cause of depression among the elderly in our society, whether they live independently, in a retirement community, in an assisted living complex or in a skilled nursing facility. The continued need of the older person for loving touch is poignantly expressed in this portion of a poem entitled, "Minnie Remembers."[8]

> How long has it been since someone touched me
> Twenty years?
> Twenty years I've been a widow
> Respected.
> Smiled at.
> But never touched.
> Never held so close that loneliness
> was blotted out.

The prescription for touch deprivation for the elderly and the ill is really quite simple. The remedy is neither time consuming nor costly. The results of touch therapy, which can be administered by almost any willing and caring person who is comfortable making conscious physical contact with another, are easily identifiable, the effects immediately noticeable.

INCREASED MOBILITY

Range of motion exercises should be left to the physical therapists trained in this area unless you are working under the auspices of, or in tandem with, such a person. However, an increase in circulation and the reduction in tension produced through the practice of gentle massage and touch techniques may well bring about subtle increases in mobility. This may be because the person being touched experiences a feeling of renewed strength or energy as a result of the focused attention. It may also be a result of the relaxation that has occurred as a result of being touched in a comforting, caring way.

I have observed lonely and less mobile elders become more inclined to feed themselves, or even to stand or walk with help after touch sessions. An increase in mobility or range of motion may also be noticed in smaller movements such as hand grasp strength or the ability of a person to reach out and pick up a cup of water or other object without help.

I remember Dad telling me that he had prayed for some help and some relief—and shortly thereafter you appeared on the scene. He always felt that you were the answer to that prayer. He enjoyed your sessions and visits very much.

LETTER FROM DAUGHTER OF RESIDENT
TO MASSAGE THERAPIST
ROSE GILMOUR

What am I supposed to do now? Where should I go? Is anybody coming to get me?

NURSING HOME RESIDENT
SITTING IN WHEELCHAIR IN HALLWAY

The touch sessions are so wonderful and give me something to look forward to. Thank you for coming!

JOSEPHINE NICHOLSON, AGE 86,
STROKE SURVIVOR

EXPERIENCE OF BEING NURTURED AND CARED FOR

Sensitive touch and gentle, caring massage is one of the most relaxing and pleasant comfort measures we can provide for others, especially for those who may be experiencing touch deprivation along with physical and emotional trauma or injury. Intentional, conscious touch is a reassuring form of physical contact and communication, a tangible act of caring. It not only feels good but it gives the receiver a sense of being nurtured and attended to, which can affect the quality of that person's life regardless of how much longer he or she continues in the physical body.

In the course of a long illness, which may include a variety of medical treatments and invasive procedures, a person can begin to feel more like scrutinized object than an individual. Those who are living with a temporary or permanent disfigurement or with physical "abnormalities" may feel unattractive and sense that others are uncomfortable or embarrassed in their presence or are repelled by the sight of their bodies. Their self-esteem may begin to degenerate along with their bodies. Respectful, attentive touch tells such people, in essence, that they are not ugly or untouchable, that they have value as human beings. If such touch is offered openly, lovingly and non-intrusively, those people will be affected by another's willingness to touch them and by that person's desire to help ease their suffering. This type of contact contributes not only to the receiver's physical comfort, but to an improved state of mind, emotional balance and overall sense of well-being. If the intention is pure and directed toward the individual, he or she will experience the touch giver's compassion and may begin to feel greater self-acceptance and self worth, becoming more "at ease" or calmer in regard to his or her physical problems and more accepting of a difficult situation.

Many of the frail elderly whom I have visited in their homes or in care facilities—especially those who receive few visitors—have fallen into a state of inertia due to extended inactivity and boredom. Regular focused touch can help break this cycle. Touch sessions provide physical and mental stimulation by increasing the circulation of oxygen and the flow of blood throughout the body, including the brain. The personal attention and human contact can boost self-esteem. When conversation is possible, verbal interaction can also stimulate brain activity. I have observed elders suddenly "come alive" and begin moving, talking and even singing after receiving one-on-one attention in the form of something as seemingly simply as hand lotioning or a back rub. I have also observed care facility residents who were labeled as "troublemakers" or incessant "whiners" become sweet and docile when touched in a sensitive, conscious and caring way.

Massage or skilled touch sessions administered over a period of time may accelerate the benefits to the receiver, yet even one short session can sometimes produce remarkable changes in a receptive patient. I once walked into a room in an extended care facility and saw a pajama-clad resident with no covers over him curled up in a fetal position on his mattress. He had oxygen tubes in his nostrils, looked very uncomfortable and seemed to be quite ill. I remember being somewhat reluctant to disturb this gentleman, as he appeared to be sleeping, yet

I was moisturizing and massaging the hands of an elderly woman I had grown particularly fond of. This sweet lady was in an advanced stage of dementia, unable to communicate with words and quite agitated the first time I met her. Over time, she had become more and more responsive to attention and touch, often smiling sweetly and occasionally venturing outside of her own private universe to speak a few coherent words before she lapsed back into making continuous repetitive sounds, her gaze unfocused and wandering. On this day, as I was applying lotion to her hands, she unexpectedly reached out and began stroking my hands! She looked at the bottle of lotion for a moment and then at my hands. I dispensed a little of the lotion into her hands and then we continued for awhile in a mutual hand lotioning and massaging session. This giving, interactive response on her part provided a wonderfully moving and memorable few moments.

AUTHOR

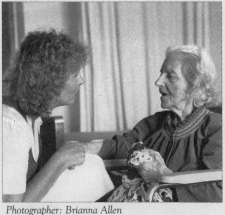

Photographer: Brianna Allen

he had requested my services and his was the last name on my list of people to see that day. He was somewhat responsive to touch, though we never made eye contact and he spoke very little during the twenty minutes or so I spent massaging his back and his extremities. Something about this man, whom I had never met before and felt quite sure I would never see again, touched my heart. At the end of our session I told him quite honestly that I was very glad to have met him and to have spent a bit of time with him. I received a telephone call from the activity director of the facility the next day telling me that, much to her amazement, she had encountered the last gentleman I'd worked with out walking in the hallway asking when he could get another massage! He left to go home a few days later.

EMOTIONAL OR ENERGY RELEASE

As most massage therapists know, intuitive and skillful touch can act as a key to unlock "stuck energy" and emotions that have been denied or held in for months, even years. As a person experiences being accepted and cared for through loving touch, as tense muscles begin to relax and the heart begins to open, it is not at all uncommon for long-repressed feelings to surface. Trembling, shaking, laughter or tears may accompany such emotional releases. There is almost always a deep sadness underlying an initial outburst of frustration or anger. At such times, we can provide a significant service to another in simply receiving whatever occurs without commenting or analyzing it. The person expressing long-denied feelings or releasing withheld emotions may suddenly feel a lightening of the body, an increase in energy, or a renewed interest in actively relating to others.

It is often easier for people to communicate with someone with whom they have no particular role to fulfill in life, someone who does not have the expectations and attachments to them that family members may have. Such people find it less difficult, perhaps, to share their deeper feelings with a person whom they have just met and may never see again than to talk about what they are experiencing with those who love them most.

The simplest acknowledgment of the reality of a situation can sometimes unleash a flood of emotion in a person who has few people to communicate with or who doesn't want to "burden" a family member. I remember well one not so elderly gentleman in an extended care facility. On the list I was given of residents I would be seeing that day, his name had a notation beside it that he'd had both legs amputated in the past year. In the course of our conversation during his neck and shoulder massage, he mentioned that his wife had died less than a year ago. I observed that he had experienced a lot of loss in a short period of time, and he began to cry as he told me some of the details of those losses.

I was once asked to look in on young man who was nearing death. His wheelchair-bound mother, who was widowed and in her seventies, took a special van every afternoon from the assisted living center where she resided to the extended care facility in another town to sit with her son who lay, no longer able to speak, dying from AIDS. This woman had watched her other four children die from various diseases

I once had a client, a rather frail-looking woman in her eighties whom I saw only once or twice a month. She spoke very little but seemed mentally aware and had a sweet and endearing smile. I usually applied lotion to her hands and arms to moisturize her dry skin and then rubbed her back and shoulders while she sat in her wheelchair. Halfway through one of our sessions, I was applying lotion with my hand shaped around the front of her arm, coming up and around the shoulder and sliding down the back of her arm to her hand. She started shaking suddenly as a wave of energy rippled through her entire body and she exclaimed in a loud, strong voice, "Ooohhh that feels sooooo good!" She continued to experience this release for several minutes.

AUTHOR

> *I had been told that the woman I'd be seeing had suffered a stroke. Shortly after our introduction, I began our session together by touching her feet. She quickly stated that she'd had a bad fall. I did not comment except to say I was sorry. I continued gently massaging her foot and leg and then went on to the other foot. I felt her begin to relax a bit physically and, after a few more minutes, she made what was obviously to her a painful confession, "It wasn't a fall; I had a stroke." She then began to relax mentally as well as physically, and to trust me with the deeper truth of her experience and her fears about recovery.*
>
> **AUTHOR**

Socializing helps to stave off depression, which is a problem common with senior citizens. Anything that stimulates the mind and keeps the neuron connections going will help.

DR STEVEN RUSSAK, GERONTOLOGIST

I've slowly learned that there is invariably at least one thing you can do: stay there. Sit and listen as someone cries. Stroke someone's arm, hold their hand, acknowledge your sorrow at their suffering. Say 'I'm sorry you're feeling bad.' Don't walk away.

ELISABETH OCHS, R.N.

and accidents over the years. I could only begin to imagine what she must be experiencing and what a toll this situation was exacting on her. She had been told that massage therapy was available for residents of the facility where her son resided but, according to the family services supervisor, she was highly resistant to the idea of anyone else touching her son.

I did not press this issue after introducing myself and instead began to gently massage her shoulders and upper back. She told me how wonderful it felt and how much she'd enjoyed the last massage she had received, seven years before during a hospital stay. Then, suddenly and rather abruptly, she wheeled her chair out into the hallway, indicating that she wanted me to follow her. She asked in somewhat urgent and hushed tones if I thought massage could actually help her son. I told her truthfully that it could not change the course of her son's disease or prolong his life but that it might help him to be more comfortable. She said rather dubiously, "Let's try it once a month then, but I can't pay you today." I did not feel that her son would be alive in a month, or even in a week! I sensed that my only opportunity to work with him was most likely the present moment, so I told her that immediate payment was not necessary and that I had some time available right then.

When I approached this woman's son, whom I judged to be in his mid-thirties, he was clutching a large teddy bear, thrashing back and forth on the bed, twisting the sheets and emitting a sound which could only be described as the kind of whimpering or whining cry a very frustrated and confused preschooler, grasping for control of his universe, might make. I placed one hand in the middle of his chest and touched his arm ever so gently and carefully, as I might a young child's. He turned and looked directly at me for several moments. His body movement and whimpering ceased and, soon, silent tears began to roll down his face. I said "It's all right," giving him the permission he perhaps could not give to himself, with his mother watching, to release his tears. A few minutes later, he turned over on his side and, like an exhausted child, went to sleep. To me, this incident was a clear example of the power of acceptance and acknowledgment.

ADDITIONAL BENEFITS

Human beings have a need to connect with other human beings. A number of studies have now revealed that, statistically speaking, people who are socially isolated tend to be less healthy. Dr. James Lynch, author of *The Broken Heart: The Medical Consequences of Loneliness* showed, for instance, that physical contact with or even the presence of another person can have a calming effect on cardiac physiology.[9]

A touch session offers someone who receives few visitors or opportunities for social interaction a chance to speak and actually be listened to. Studies have shown increased activity in the brain during stimulation through touch, and caring touch can open the door for an expression of thoughts and feelings that may have been withheld for months or even years.

It may take repeated visits or touch sessions to build trust and rapport with a person, especially if that person is naturally reticent or suspicious. I can recall several times when I've spent half-a-dozen sessions with someone, in relative silence, before he or she spoke directly to me or made an effort to communicate verbally.

I have met aged residents in care facilities who have simply outlived their friends and what few family members they may have had, or whose family consists of one or two relatives who live far away. I have known of residents who went months or even years without a visitor from the outside world other than a Salvation Army volunteer at Christmas time. Other residents may be socially shy or withdrawn and are not easily persuaded to leave their rooms or to participate in group activities that are offered. For such people, opportunities for interactions that are not task or treatment oriented or for diagnostic purposes may be few and far between.

In introducing myself for the first time to a person within the care facility setting, I have sometimes been greeted, initially with suspicion ("What do you want from me?") or resignation ("What do you need me to do now?"). Such responses are understandable since most residents are used to being visited by people with specific tasks or goals. The recreational therapist, the speech therapist, the physical therapist, the social worker, the occupational therapist, and so on, each have a specific responsibility in relation to the resident: each one has a program, plan or task to carry out and a limited amount of time to spend with each person. Family members who do visit may also have their own agendas. In addition, their interactions with the resident are taking place within life-long habits or relationship dynamics that may affect the quality of their visits with an aging loved one or limit their capacity to be present in an unconditional way.

Nursing and administrative staff are, unfortunately, often way too busy and burdened to spend time "just" getting to know the residents better as one might with a neighbor or new friend. I was stunned by something a retired nurse told me a few years ago. She said that a nursing supervisor at the hospital where she had last worked told her entire staff one day, "Don't ever look your patients in the eye because then they'll want to talk to you." I am convinced that some elderly residents of care facilities stop talking simply because there is no one to listen to what they may have to say. I think that imaginary friends and the one-sided conversations which are carried out with those friends are sometimes the result of loneliness rather than a psychiatric problem.

The verbal interaction and socialization afforded by focused, one-on-one attention can be as nourishing, and sometimes as important, as a nutritionally balanced meal, especially to the aged. I am certain that many of the people I see in convalescent facilities and homes for the aged benefit as much from the conversations we have, and from being listened to, as they do from the physical contact they usually receive during our sessions.

I remember a nursing home resident who always responded positively to my presence and seemed to enjoy being touched. She made eye contact with me and smiled, her body relaxed, and she sometimes sighed audibly, yet she never spoke. I never tried to force a conversation. It didn't seem necessary to our interaction. One day, as I was gently massaging one of her shoulders and looking into her eyes, she suddenly said, "It's so boring in here." Smiling, I asked her what kinds of things she enjoyed doing before coming to her present address; and in the next fifteen minutes, with little prodding from me, she talked almost nonstop, painting a vivid picture of her former life.

AUTHOR

There is hunger for ordinary bread, and there is hunger for love, for kindness, for thoughfulness.

MOTHER THERESA

One patient I remember well just lived for her massage and she guided me and told me just what she wanted. To be able to help a patient relax by simply touching them and being with them is a wonderful thing to be able to do... it's rewarding for me.

DOROTHY CHAKNOVA, C.M.T.

May God establish the works of my hands and may the works of my hands establish God.

JEWISH SABBATH SERVICE

Knowing I'm able to give a little spark, just a little bit of happiness and love through just a gentle touch is so beneficial to me. It's instant gratification.

DEANNA MATTHEWS, C.M.T.

BENEFITS FOR THE GIVER OF TOUCH

I once noticed a title on a bookstore shelf, *The Healing Power of Doing Good*. It is now known that helping others enhances one's own health, physically and psychologically. Dr. Herbert Benson, author of *The Relaxation Response*, said that he might well prescribe volunteerism as a way to reduce stress. An act of selfless giving can raise self-esteem, boost energy, help us lead more productive lives, and even add years to a lifetime!

Ancient wisdom also suggests that giving to others is a gift to the self. Jesus said that "It is more blessed to give than to receive." Eastern religions teach that generosity and kindness to others brings the

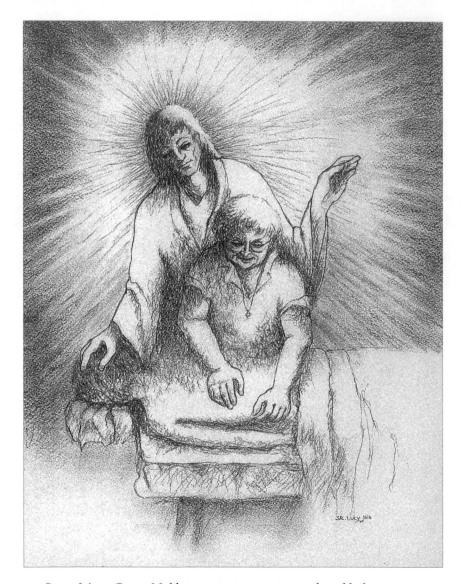

Sister Mary Grace Noble gave a massage to another elderly sister in her order of nuns. At the end of their session, Sister Lucy told her that she had felt Christ's hands touching her and giving her comfort while Sister Mary Grace was giving her the massage. She sketched this drawing to illustrate her experience.

greatest happiness, purifying the heart and mind; and that inner tranquility and strength come from the development of love and compassion.

Using our hands to nurture and comfort, making skin-to-skin contact conscious, tends to heighten our sense of touch, making us more sensitive, not only to other's bodies but to our own bodies, and it helps us understand and acknowledge our own need for nurturing and love. It helps us develop compassion for ourselves as well as compassion for others.

Caring for the elderly and the ill, whether that task is a chosen profession, a volunteer activity, or a role that we unexpectedly inherit, can be both challenging and enlightening. It may catapult us into unfamiliar territory, requiring us to navigate in uncharted terrain as we endeavor to provide life-sustaining assistance and relief to those with whom we are sharing life's journey.

The act of caring for others reminds us of how much we actually have to give. As we dive deeper into our pool of resources in order to meet the rigorous demands and responsibilities of caregiving, we may discover strengths and abilities we did not know we possessed.

Opening our hearts to others helps us identify ways in which we might ease the suffering of our fellow human beings. It informs us of our kinship with others, highlights our interdependence and enables us to experience the joy of our intrinsic connection. Including conscious and nurturing physical contact in the act of caregiving provides us with a specific vehicle for service, and an avenue for expressing our innate generosity.

Choosing to be consciously *present with* and *attentive to* another human being creates a space for us to experience what is actually true in regard to that individual. When we follow our instinctive impulses to reach out in merciful kindness and care for another, we are acting from a level of beingness that is close to our own true nature. Anytime we come out of our self-ness by deepening our contact with others, we have an opportunity to experience who we really are.

Spending time with the dying teaches us how to be in the presence of suffering and to keep our hearts open instead of shutting down, turning away or denying the pain we experience in ourselves and in others. In staying open we may experience the illusion of separateness dissolving.

The most significant benefit of a massage or touch practice that specializes in relating to the elderly and the seriously ill may be simply getting to know another human being whom we otherwise would never have met. Any time we truly open our hearts to others, a part of who we are is reflected back to us and our vision is thus expanded. The personal bond that is created out of the intimate interaction in a touch session is of immeasurable benefit because it is always in the context of relationship that true healing and evolution can occur.

J, the resident that reminds me so much of my grandpa, brought me to tears as I left his room the first time I met him. I walked out of his room filled with joy and a "this is why I do this" feeling. When I first went in, he was sitting in his Lazy Boy with his walker in front of the chair. I moved the walker so he could put his feet up for a massage. When I was finished, I put the chair back down and returned the walker to the front of his chair, like it had been when I got there. I was putting stuff back in my bag and saw he was struggling to stand up. I picked up my bag and said "Where are you headed?" and started to add that I'd walk along with him, when it became apparent that he was just standing up because a lady was leaving. Who does THAT anymore?!

KIM PALKA, L.M.T.

My religion is very simple – my religion is kindness.

DALAI LAMA

Man becomes great exactly in the degree to which he works for the welfare of his fellow men.

MAHATMA GANDHI

I have been an R.N. for six years and a massage therapist for three years. Many people ask me why I wanted to become a massage therapist. Until your lecture I always struggled for an answer. I was reminded of a very powerful experience I had during nursing school. I was working at a local hospital for the summer halfway through my training. There was an older gentleman who was a patient... Arthritis had taken hold of his hands, I don't think he could see well and he was, generally speaking, very ill. Many of the nurses on the floor didn't want to work with him because he was "too demanding." As you can guess the young "nurse wannabe" was frequently assigned to him. Funny thing was, I didn't think he was demanding. He was a man in his eighties who was spending many weeks in a hospital room regularly hooked up to a dialysis machine for three or four hours at a time. His family visited regularly and he very much enjoyed company... One night he had dinner in his room with his son. It was a busy night on the floor... After dinner when this gentleman asked the nurse assigned to him if she would sit with him... and she told him she "didn't have time," I went to ask my supervisor if I could go sit with Carl and she said that would be fine. I walked down to his room (about five minutes had passed) and when I approached him, I realized he had passed away. I was filled with emotion, anger that I was unable to say good-bye, sadness that he was alone at that time when he obviously didn't want to be, and relief that he was finally free of his pain and suffering.

I have recalled this event many times since then, and I suspect it will always be a reminder of how important a few minutes can be to a person. I think I realized during that summer I wasn't going to be what I wanted to be if I was just a nurse. What I wanted was to be a nurse of years past when the patient was more important than the paperwork.

Jennifer Purcell, Spokane, Washington

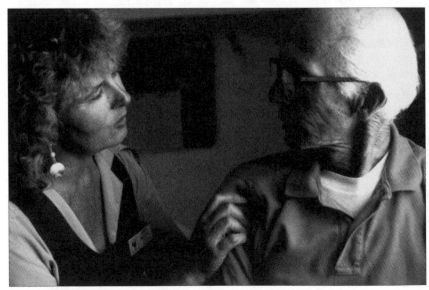

Photographer: Brock Palmer

Karmic Touch

I t was more than thirty years after my grandparents rescued me from my mother's abusive neglect when my interest in touch led me to begin taking bodywork classes, and I had the opportunity to offer my grandmother a massage. By this time she'd lost both her breasts to cancer and my grandfather to heart disease. She was well into her eighties and her spirit was as alive and sparkling as ever but her body was beginning to show signs of frailty. She had gotten on an airplane

and flown up to northern California to visit me during a somewhat difficult period in my life when I had enrolled in graduate school and was living with my two young children in a rented house.

My grandmother was always enthusiastic about whatever I was doing and when I told her about my extracurricular massage classes, she lent me her body to practice on without hesitation. Since I didn't yet own a massage table, I had her lie down on the bed with the firmest mattress, and I knelt on my knees to give her a back and shoulder massage. Her body felt so utterly different from those of my fellow

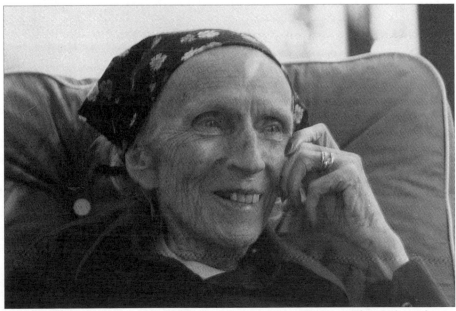

Photographer: unknown

My father was bedridden and suffering from a fistula. My duties consisted mostly of dressing the wound and giving my father his medicine. Every night I massaged his legs and retired only when he asked me to do so or after he had fallen asleep... I loved to do this service.

MAHATMA GHANDI, IN *AUTOBIOGRAPHY*

My mother became like an altar, the focus of our loving attention, the place where we sat for periods in silence, spoke special words, and physically cared for her as one would care for anything sacred and loved... Once I was looking at her as she slept and I remembered a specific time when I was about six and had woken up in the middle of the night. I called out for her... and she came to me. As I remembered this, tears came to my eyes as I realized the beautiful simplicity of her response. After she awoke I said to her, 'While you were sleeping, I remembered a time when I was six. I called out for you in the middle of the night, and... you came. She was weak at this stage, but she heard me. She just closed her eyes and smiled a little smile. There was nothing more to say.

Lawrence Noyes

I remember my mother's swollen and gnarled fingers, able to express so much through her loving touch and creativity. My parents were my initial teachers of sacred touch.

EVELYN M. GERARDO, L.M.T.,
CHAPLAIN

---

students in class! As my hands moved down her back, I felt bones instead of muscles; and the wrinkles and the thinness of her skin startled me. My newly acquired confidence in my massage skills was slightly shaken but my heart took over.

From a technical point of view it was certainly not the best massage I ever gave, yet it was undoubtedly one of the most loving and most gratifying. As I stroked the familiar freckled, sun-kissed arms that had hugged and held me, touched the hands that had fed and bathed and lifted me into bed night after night so many years before, I looked into my grandmother's smiling eyes, and felt an immense gratitude. It sanctified something in our relationship for me to be able to offer myself in service to her in that particular way. It was an inexpressible gift to me to be able to give back in some small measure, even for those few minutes, a tiny piece of what she had given me through the loving, hands-on care that had helped to heal my body and my spirit so long ago.

Years later, when I was making a living providing touch services to the elderly and the ill, a woman telephoned and asked me to come to see her mother, whom she was caring for in her home. Her mother had been living with Alzheimer's disease for some years and was nearing death. When I arrived, the cheerful yet rather fatigued-looking woman who had called thanked me for coming and took me immediately into the room where her mother lay in a hospital bed, her eyes open but unfocused. She went directly to the bed, leaned over her mother and began softly stroking her cheek. 'Isn't my mother beautiful?' she said, smiling. I could, indeed, see the beauty of the older woman, reflected in the loving eyes of her daughter. The daughter began talking about what a wonderful person her mother was (not had once been but in the present tense) and she continued to touch her mother's body, stroking her hair, kissing her on the cheek and holding her hand in both of hers. She told me that she had quit her job in order to take care of her mother and that she hoped to keep her at home until her death. She acknowledged that it was a financial sacrifice and that the full-time caregiving was hard work. She said that she was tired much of the time, yet she couldn't see doing it any other way after all her mother had done for her. I thought to myself that this mother must have been a very loving parent and that she had created good karma for herself by the way she raised her daughter. I thought how lucky both women were to have this time together and to have an opportunity to complete their cycle of caregiving with each other.

One way of looking at the concept of karma is seeing it as an opportunity to give back or return what we have been given. An opportunity for this kind of fulfillment exists when we have the good fortune to help care for our aging parents or grandparents as they near the end of their lives.

Not long after his mother's death from cancer, I sat with a good friend of mine as he reminisced about his last days with her. I was particularly struck by how the experience of helping with her physical care had affected him.

As one of her caregivers, I fed her and gave her drinks and made her comfortable. Once while feeding her I realized that this was the first time I had ever physically served her, ever served her body directly. The whole karmic situation struck me as enormously unbalanced. When I thought of all the diapers of mine she had changed, all the meals she had made for me, the sicknesses she had nursed me through, all the direct physical support she had given me, it all seemed... stunning... the imbalance of it all. She had given me and my body so much attention for so many years when I was young, and now I had only a few weeks to return the favor.

I felt honored and fortunate to be able to touch her, to hold her hand, wipe her forehead, even to clean her up after she used the bedpan. Under these circumstances there is something sacred about this, that I think mothers know when caring for an infant. On the surface, it sounds unpleasant, even disgusting, but under circumstances of unconditional love and respect, a kind of transformation makes it into a sacred event.[10]

When my father-in-law underwent surgery to remove part of a cancerous lung, he insisted on going back to his apartment when he was released from the hospital rather than coming to our home or going to someone else's to recuperate. My husband went over daily to change his bandages, help him bathe and dress and do whatever else needed to be done to support his father's healing. My husband had no nursing experience but his love for his father guided his hands. The two adult men already had a close intellectual bond and friendship, yet this circumstance created a new dimension in their relationship.

I felt really grateful that I could do something for my father as he had done for me. It increased the physical intimacy between us, not necessarily the emotional or psychic intimacy but the physical intimacy. I remember acutely him being surprised that I was instantly willing to do something that he needed done, as if he was surprised that I loved him that much.[11]

Some years ago, I was asked to address a group of men and women caring for parents or spouses with Alzheimer's disease. I listened as various people shared their struggles and their feelings; and I spoke informally about the benefits of skilled touch and massage for those living with Alzheimer's, as well as for men and women such as themselves who had taken on the challenge of caring for their loved ones. At the end of the hour, the regular facilitator of the group asked if she could tell me something about herself and her father. She said it had to do with touch and that it was the most intimate moment she had ever shared with father. As she spoke, I was moved and inspired both by the words and by the depth of feeling that recalling the experience evoked in her. I asked her if she would write down what she had shared with me. I was pleased when her expanded story arrived in the mail a few weeks later.

Susan wrote eloquently about her father's voracious appetite for life, his vitality, his love of books, music, sports and politics, his passion for playing the piano. Her father had been diagnosed with lymphoma two years prior to being hospitalized for a spleenectomy. While he was still in the hospital, recovering from what she called a successful and uneventful surgery, her father suffered a heart attack. He

...the most special part of my trip was spending a few hours each day with my dad in the nursing home. I gave gentle touch massages to him and several others there and their response was so wonderful. I wasn't sure how my dad would react but he softened around the whole process and just calmed down and relaxed. Before he had been quite agitated and restless. It was so wonderful to see this change.

MARY SINGLETARY, C.M.T.

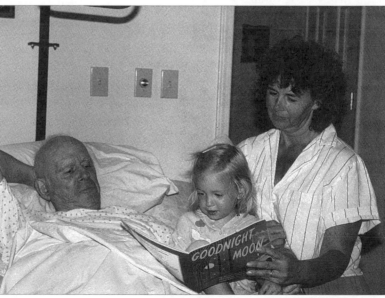

Photographer: Barry Barankin

His last few months in the nursing home my grandfather slowly stopped eating or responding to much of anything. I had been very close to him growing up but we were later estranged for some years and separated by distance as well. I went to visit him shortly before he died. I touched him and was able to get him to drink some liquids and to eat. I fed him one of his last meals. It felt good that in our last encounter he responded to me. It was a really good experience.

SALLY REGAN

My mother, a proud and stoic New Englander was quite ill with emphysema at age 81 and did not want help – except from her daughter. I changed her diapers, rubbed her back, fed her, held her hands… I had never seen my mother naked until this time. I knew her dignity was very important to her so I remained respectful… eventually she had to be hospitalized and then she slipped into a coma. As the end drew near, her breathing became very soft. My brothers and I were each holding a part of her body when a miracle occurred. She spoke to us and said "I love you all" and then peacefully took her last breath… we were all amazed. We had thought she was not aware we were even there.

PAM WILLIAMS

actually died in that moment, of congestive heart failure, and was brought back to life by the "Code Blue" staff who revived him by pounding his chest, breaking at least two ribs, and applying "jump paddles" to his heart.

In intensive care a respirator was put down his throat and his arms and legs were restrained so he couldn't grab the respirator and other assorted tubes which were stuck in every orifice of his body. My proud and dignified Father was reduced to trying to communicate by mouthing words or valiantly attempting to scribble his thoughts on a yellow pad of paper.[12]

In her letter, Susan went on to describe how excruciating it was for her to watch her father's efforts to communicate. She wrote about how relieved and buoyed everyone was when her father was taken off the life-support apparatus and able to breathe on his own. Susan then related an experience that she described as "profound and moving."

A wonderful male nurse named Mark Lamaroux asked my Father if he would like a shave. My Father said that would be wonderful and Mark went to work. In the very busy and serious atmosphere of the intensive care unit, Mark tenderly felt Dad's face for blemishes or moles, explaining that he didn't want to nick or cut him… I watched this gentle, compassionate man adeptly shave my Father's face, all the while speaking softly and assuredly to my fragile Father. That loving act of shaving my Dad totally restored him, my stepmother and me.[13]

A few weeks later, watching her father languishing in his hospital bed, and longing to do something for him, Susan remembered what a catharsis the shave had been.

I approached a nurse about shaving him. 'You can do it,' she replied brusquely. She didn't have the inclination or time. So with that she handed me the plastic razor, wash rag, towel, miniature container of shaving cream and promptly disappeared. To tell you the truth I was rather terrified. Not only had I never shaved anyone in my life I was afraid I'd hurt Dad. But at that moment I realized that giving to my Father was more important and pressing than my fears and doubts about my own ability to do it…During his three weeks of hospitalization I had stolen countless looks at my Father's face and body when he was sleeping. I had studied him like a map. I rubbed the shaving cream all over his face. He seemed totally at ease. I was still nervous but determined to succeed. I made many trips to the bathroom sink to replenish the warm water. By the time I finished I don't think I cut him but his hospital gown was soaked on the top. I most certainly had not given him a smooth shave but I think I had soothed his soul for those minutes. I was touching him in a way I never had before. I was serving him…Dad died at home some days later…If had he died in the hospital right after his heart attack he and I would have been deprived of one of the most moving experiences of my life.[14]

When the roles that we are used to playing and which we take for granted in life are reversed and a person whom we have depended on all our lives to protect us, advise us and care for us suddenly needs taking care of himself or needs us to guide and protect her, it can be startling for both parties. Such role reversals are not always accepted easily or without resentment. The problems in the relationship do not magically disappear when the caregiving role reverses. In fact sometimes they escalate. Yet the new way of relating can also serve to create fresh insights and deeper understanding. Even in the midst of the hardship that such a shift may present, fences are often mended and old hurts may be healed.

The opportunity to participate in the physical act of caring for someone who has once cared for us may help us learn to appreciate how much was given, how many ways there are to care. It may also assist us in reordering priorities and simplifying our relationships. Author and physician Rachel Naomi Remen passes on a story from a talk she gave about her work with people with cancer to a group of women physicians:

One of the physicians talked about caring for her dying mother when she was nineteen years old. She had expected a great deal less of herself then. At first she had driven her mother to her doctor's appointments, shopped for food, and run errands. As her mother grew weaker, she had prepared tempting meals and cleaned the house. When her mother stopped eating, she had listened to her and read to her for hours. When her mother slipped into coma, she had changed her sheets, bathed her and rubbed her back with lotion. There always seemed to be something more to do. A way to care. These ways became simpler and simpler. "In the end," she told us, "I just held her and sang."[15]

Another process that can unfold in what one might describe as karmic caregiving is a dissolving of the roles altogether. There may come a time when we can let go of our attachment to the role or when all guises disappear. There is no parent, no child, no helper, no one needing help. There are no buried grudges, no unforgiven hurts, no lingering mistrust. There are just two individuals caught up in the perplexities of life, inextricably bound together by genetics or fate and by their shared humanity. Or perhaps, in a moment of Grace, there is simply no separation at all.

I once read a very moving story, which illustrates the potential for healing that occurs when we are able to go beyond familiar relationship models and roles and allow ourselves to simply be present with another individual.

A woman whose father is near death tells of being called to come when his condition worsens. She goes directly from the airport to the hospital and then to her father's room. Seeing a very old, very pale, thin man in the bed, she thinks she has entered the wrong room and then suddenly understands that she has not recognized her own father.

Thank God he was asleep. All I could do was sit next to him and try to get past this image before he woke up and saw my shock. I had to look through him and find something beside this astonishing appearance of a father I could barely recognize physically. By the time he awoke, I'd gotten part of the way. But we were still quite uncomfortable with one another. There was still this sense of distance. We both could feel it. It was very painful. We both were self-conscious.[16]

Several days later as this woman is sitting beside her sleeping father, she suddenly thinks of something Mother Theresa once said, describing the lepers she cared for as "Christ in all his distressing disguises" and she is able to see her father behind his disguise, as a child of God. She experiences her own identity as being the same as his identity. This occurrence precipitates a different relationship with her father, unlike anything she has known before.

At that point he woke up and looked at me and said, "Hi." And I looked at him and said, "Hi." For the remaining months of his life we were totally at peace and comfortable together. No more self-consciousness. No unfinished business. I usually seemed to know just what was needed. I could feed him, shave him, bathe him, hold him up to fix the pillows—all these very intimate things that had been so hard for me earlier.

In a way, this was my father's final gift to me: the chance to see him as something more than my father; the chance to see the common identity of spirit we both shared; the chance to see just how much that makes possible in the way of love and comfort. And I feel I can call on it now with anyone else.[17]

As a teacher of mine once said, "When you let go of everything only the truth remains." It is in such moments that two souls can meet in a place beyond chosen identities, roles and dualities, where even time and space do not exist.

The Power of Touch in Facility Care

STRESS OF ADJUSTMENT TO GROUP COMMUNITY

In the past quarter century, the number of people over age sixty-five has increased by more than 55 percent, making that group of individuals the fastest growing segment of our society. As the "baby boomers" age and life spans increase, the number of people with chronic illnesses or disabilities that require long-term healthcare services is also increasing.

More people are living longer than ever before in our history. Thanks to the medical science that has extended their lives, many elders with late onset diseases require more professional attention than family-based custodial care can provide. This year, it is estimated that nine million older Americans will need extended healthcare.

At one time, transfer to a nursing or convalescent home after a period of hospitalization was primarily for rehabilitation or for continued recovery after an accident, surgical procedure or acute illness. Often the patient would complete his or her recovery at home, being cared for by a family member or close friend. In today's society, that process is no longer the norm. Increasing frailty in the aging process, a debilitating disease or a chronic illness, along with one or more of following circumstances usually precipitates a move into some type of extended healthcare facility:

A colleague of mine, a psychiatrist, had been working for three years with a severely burned woman, trying to teach her that she was lovable in spite of her scars. After hearing me lecture... the next time the woman came in, he went over and hugged her. He said she improved more with that hug than with three years of therapy.

DR. BERNIE SIEGEL

When I arrived at the Respite Center that day I noticed that one of the more active participants in the program was uncharacteristically quiet and withdrawn. When I sat down next to her wheelchair and put my attention on her, she seemed to be on the verge of tears. I asked her what was wrong. As the tears spilled over onto her face, she whispered "I don't live in my house anymore." Without warning, according to her, her daughters had moved her into "one of those facilities," telling her she would be there for a few days. She had soon discovered that the move was to be permanent and was struggling to accept her new circumstance. She spoke of the other woman in the room not liking her and complaining about her snoring and then said plaintively, "but she snores too!

AUTHOR

The work I do with the residents has been so rewarding... I work with residents who have had strokes, Parkinson's, Huntington's disease, dementia, Alzheimer's and general senility... Some of the residents have no or very few contacts with the outside world. Some have very little contact with their families. They are touched by the nurses, doctors and C.N.A.'s but the touch they receive from me is something special.

MICKY ANDERSON, L.M.T.

- hospitalization that requires continued medical attention
- an inability to care for oneself safely
- specialized care needed is too expensive or too difficult for family members
- a lack of family caregivers to provide needed care
- caregiver burnout
- death of spouse or other caregiver

The relocation may require moving out of a long-established residence and giving up a lifetime of material possessions, tangible symbols and reminders of one's past, which are put into storage, sold or distributed among family members.

While the move into a care facility may be necessary and can have positive effects or eventual outcomes, inherent in such a transition are additional deprivations such as the loss of

- familiar environment, activities and resources
- established routines
- social relationships
- personal space
- privacy
- community structure and support
- decreased contact with the outside world

Whether the person being relocated recognizes the necessity of the move and consciously chooses to make the change, or the person is encouraged or even pressured by loved ones to do so, the transition is often fraught with difficulties, especially at the onset, for everyone involved. Family members may not be certain they are doing the right thing and are perhaps plagued by feelings of guilt or anxiety. The new resident finds him or herself suddenly relegated to a different bed in an unfamiliar and possibly much smaller living space. There may be little or no room for treasured and familiar objects. The person is often "placed" in a room with one, two or even three people he or she has never met before and may have little in common with. Real privacy is minimal. It is seldom quiet.

Some facility residents are stroke survivors whose self-image has eroded in their struggle to adapt to functional limitations. Some may be confronting life-threatening diseases such as cancer or AIDS. Over 50 percent have some form of dementia. Many have more than one condition or disease and are taking multiple medications.

I have known a number of care facility residents who have outlived friends and even family members. Changes in visual acuity and other physical impairments sometimes curtail leisure activities that once helped pass the time. I remember one mentally alert woman in her nineties, who had been climbing mountains in her eighties and who enjoyed our conversations as much as her massage during our sessions, saying to me, "If they'd just let me go out and walk five or ten miles I'd be fine."

Touch becomes increasingly important for those in extended care homes who receive few visitors from the outside world. Though their basic needs are met, these women and men can remain starved for the nourishment that comes through one-on-one attention and skin-to-skin human contact.

Quality of Life Issues

Being touched in a way that is nurturing, relaxing and pleasurable is an experience largely denied the aged and the ill in our culture and this is particularly true for the men and women who are living out their lives in healthcare facilities. At first glance, it may seem as if nursing home residents are receiving a lot of physical contact. However, most of that physical contact comes during daily care activities such as bathing or dressing or during specific, and sometimes invasive, medical procedures. Such touch is not always conscious nor is it intentionally provided as an effort to enhance quality of life, and some residents receive very little one-on-one, unconditional attention in the form of touch.

Skilled touch is particularly adaptable to comfort care in the nursing home environment. Massage is well known for its ability to reduce muscular tension, relieve minor aches and pains, increase circulation and induce a relaxation response in the body. Recent research indicates that massage can boost the immune system, a discovery that has far reaching implications in the search for ways to ward off opportunistic infections in those with compromised immune systems. It is now thought that massage may stimulate the release of endorphins, the body's natural painkillers, into the brain and nervous system. The physiological reaction to caring touch, it is currently postulated, helps rebalance the flow of nerve chemicals within the brain called neurotransmitters, which may be responsible for the feelings of well-being or euphoria which often follow a massage or touch session.[18]

In addition to the physical benefits of a body-based therapy such as massage, unconditional and intentional touch can have significant psychosocial benefits for short or long-term residents of care facilities providing them with

- skin-to-skin contact
- one-on-one attention
- tactile and sensory stimulation
- an opportunity for social interaction
- comfort
- nurturing
- reassurance
- pleasure

Touch is a universal language. As such, it assists in reinforcing and facilitating communication with those who are less verbal, and with those who may have difficulty expressing themselves or understanding spoken language. It can be a primary means of communicating with those who are nonverbal.

Skillfully applied, compassionate, caring touch helps address quality of life issues common in facility care such as

- touch deprivation
- loneliness
- feelings of isolation
- low self-esteem
- anxiety

I never had a massage before. It was so relaxing!

ANNA PERRET, NURSING HOME RESIDENT, AGE 98.

Think about touch in your own life. If you go to the doctor and you have your blood pressure checked or your ears checked, you are being touched but it's not the same as when you go home and your spouse hugs you and massages your shoulders, or your child jumps into your arms and kisses you. That's a totally different type of touch that we all need in our lives. We all know how good that feels in our own lives and if we thought about what it would be like if we didn't have that kind of loving touch, we would better understand what it is like for those residents and how very important that kind of touch is. Most of our clients tend to be touch deprived. They may receive touch from the caregivers if they're getting assistance bathing, dressing, may receive some form of touch when they're eating but that's not the same as a loving touch, as a hug or a massage, a focused, gentle touch. And they need that and when they're deprived of that you'll know and when somebody's getting that touch you'll know it. It totally changes the person.

BRIANNA ALLEN, CARE FACILITY DIRECTOR

We were taught in nursing school to give an evening backrub and settle patients in for, hopefully, a good night's sleep... all of our medical approaches have become so high-tech that we have lost some of the healing aspects of the caring, nurturing component of healthcare that are so important.

MARIAN WILLIAMS, R.N., C.M.T.

Everyone acknowledges the fact that infants and young children need to be touched, but our culture fails to understand that we never outgrow the need for touch.

HELEN CAMPBELL, C.M.T.

The look on the faces of the residents when I walk in their room is priceless. Some are able to talk and some are not. Whether they can say it or not, I know they are happy to see me. I get just as much benefit from this experience as they do.

MICKY ANDERSON, L.M.T.

A lovely young lady just came to my room and do you know, she listened to me, she touched me and she didn't tell me I was old!

NURSING HOME RESIDENT AFTER VISIT
FROM WORKSHOP PARTICIPANT

- boredom
- depression
- lethargy

Skilled touch can be utilized in dealing with challenging behaviors such as

- restlessness
- wandering
- agitation
- fearfulness
- withdrawal

Years ago, nurses were taught how to give back massages, instead of pills, to help lull their patients into restful sleep at bedtime. Unfortunately, most nurses these days are kept so busy dispensing pain-reducing and sleep-inducing medications that they have no time to give back rubs or visit with their charges.

A retired nurse I know thinks that the nursing profession has become more about pills and paperwork than about compassionate care. She says that she was glad to retire so she could become a volunteer and get back to doing the things she was trained to do in nursing school such as giving back rubs to help people relax.

In his now classic book on touch, author Ashley Montagu states that "touching as a therapeutic event is not as simple as a mechanical procedure or a drug, because it is, above all, an act of communication."[19] Montagu believed that the need for tactile stimulation increases as a person ages. And yet the aged are so often deprived of the one thing that can assuage isolation and "communicate loved, trust, affection and warmth."[20]

NEED FOR TOUCH THROUGHOUT THE LIFE CYCLE

Much has been made of the fact that human contact in the form of touch is crucial during the early stages of life. Some now famous research, which was carried out on institutionalized infants over fifty years ago, showed that babies who were not held and cuddled lost interest in eating, became emaciated and failed to thrive. Researchers concluded that the stimulation of touch was vital to life and health. More recently, Dr. Tiffany Field, Director of the Touch Research Institute and a psychology professor at the University of Miami Medical School, has conducted several research studies on the effects of massage on infants. She found that babies who received massage during their first few days of life gained weight and developed nearly twice as quickly as the babies who were not being massaged.[21]

Doesn't it stand to reason that touch is as essential at the end of the life cycle—when we are again vulnerable, fragile and dependent on others for our care—as it is at the beginning of our lives? I have encountered residents in the hallways and doorways of nursing homes reaching out their arms and, quite literally, crying to be touched, longing for contact and for acknowledgment of the continued worth of their existence.

An unpublished report from a case study conducted by Christine Gruschke, Nurse Consultant for Beverly Health and Rehabilitation Services, Inc. (1997) showed a tremendous improvement in mood and anxiety levels in residents receiving massage once a week for an average of three months in a Florida nursing home. Perhaps most noteworthy was the documented reduction in medications (representing a significant financial savings) taken for pain management for many of the twenty-one residents in this particular study.

A study conducted by the Foundation for Long Term Care, Inc. in Albany, New York in 1997–98 on 130 nursing home residents with dementia showed that attentive touch sessions administered several times a week had a positive impact on sleep patterns. Staff members in the ten nursing homes that participated in the project felt that the attentive touch sessions were beneficial.

It is my belief that the aged among us who are confined to care facilities and who continue to be touch deprived begin to experience a diminishing quality of life, a lessening of their desire to interact with others and a weakening of what may already be a fragile relationship with reality. Feelings of isolation and abandonment can escalate, contributing to inertia and depression which, in turn, can lead to a "failure to thrive" syndrome.

Skilled touch is a cost-effective, non-pharmacological technique for reducing stress and enhancing quality of life for the elderly and ill in care facility environments. Touch gives pleasure, nourishment,

Touching is marvelous because that's the stuff that is beyond the therapy and all the hygiene things that you have to go through, getting them out of bed and so on... If you leave them alone, they're just sitting there waiting to die... She's a human being, she's alive, she breathes, and she deserves some respect, some dignity.

JACK ZANETTE, SON OF
NURSING HOME RESIDENT

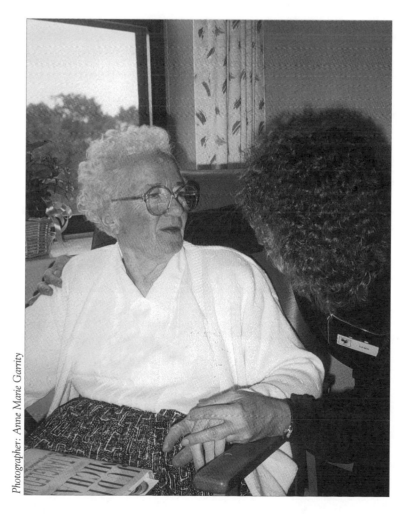

Photographer: Anne Marie Garrity

I went into L's room and she was in her wheelchair, her head and neck arched way back and her arms crossed tight into her chest. She was breathing with difficulty and making occasional agitated-type sounds. I put my hands on her shoulders, told her who I was and that I was going to spend a few minutes with her. I did some cranial polarity holds and I talked to her every so often. About ten minutes into the session she took a huge breath and put her arms partway down. When I left after twenty minutes her hands were in her lap and she was breathing much better. I went along to the next person and then a little after noon I was in the administrator's office because all the residents were at lunch, an aide came in and said that when she was starting to feed L, she took two deep breaths and died. I then found out that she had been diagnosed with metastatic colon cancer and that she'd been "trying to die for a week now."

Kim Palka, L.M.T.

warmth and comfort. It offers reassurance to those who are traumatized, lonely and afraid and helps restore feelings of self-esteem and self-worth. Touch is a powerful acknowledgment to the individual that, regardless of the condition of his or her physical body or mental state, that person still has value. It lets that person know that someone cares and that he or she is not alone.

RESOURCES

The Touch Research Institute offers published studies free of charge upon request. You can contact the Institute through the University of Miami School of Medicine, Dept. of Pediatrics, P.O. Box 01620 (D-820), Miami, FL 33101. Phone: 305-547-6781. Fax: 305-243-6488.

The Power of Touch in Alzheimer's/ Dementia Care

MEMORY LOSS

Many people over the age of fifty have trouble remembering things occasionally. Forgetfulness is thought to be a normal part of aging. Nearly everyone experiences the minor frustration of being unable to retrieve the right word from time to time or of misplacing objects such as pens or glasses. I once heard a speaker talk about the difference between this type of normal forgetfulness and a memory lapse that might be associated with a disease such as Alzheimer's. He said that if you are looking for your reading or sunglasses and they are propped on the top of your head, then you are probably experiencing what has become popularly known as a "senior moment." If, however, your bifocals are on your face and you think you have never worn glasses, that is likely a signal of a more serious problem.

Age-associated forgetfulness and memory losses in the beginning stages of various dementia-related diseases may seem confusingly similar. One difference is that the memory loss associated with Alzheimer's tends to progress more rapidly, last longer and soon become more apparent to family and friends. The chart on the next page, adapted from *Care of Alzheimer's Patients: A Manual for Nursing Home Staff* by Lisa P. Gwyther summarizes the difference between Alzheimer's disease and age-associated memory failures and how each affects one's life.

As a group, people with dementia can be spontaneous, funny and loving, and that's the reward. It's also very satisfying to be part of a movement to help maintain the quality of life for a group of people who not long ago were warehoused or generally written-off.

NORA REUTER, MUSIC THERAPIST

DIFFERENCES BETWEEN PEOPLE WITH ALZHEIMER'S DISEASE AND AGE-ASSOCIATED MEMORY LOSS

Person	with Alzheimer's Disease	with Age-associated Memory Loss
forgets	whole experience	part of experience
remembers later	rarely	often
follows verbal or written directions	gradually cannot	usually can
can use notes	gradually cannot	usually can
able to care for self	gradually unable	usually able

DEMENTIAS DEFINED AND DIFFERENTIATED

Dementia, a term applied in reference to a group of symptoms, is usually defined as a loss of intellectual capacities such as thinking, reasoning and remembering that is severe enough to interfere with a person's day-to-day functioning. The causes and rate of progression of dementias vary. There are more than seventy different causes of dementia of which Alzheimer's disease is now known to be the most common, accounting for approximately three-quarters of all cases.[22] Other diseases that may include an irreversible dementia component are

- Multi-Infarct or Vascular Dementia (MID)
- Pick's disease
- Creutzfeldt-Jakob disease
- Huntington's disease
- Parkinson's disease
- ALS (Lou Gehrig's disease)
- MS (Multiple Sclerosis)
- Lewy Body Dementia

Some people have a combination of Alzheimer's and Vascular Dementia. Alzheimer's, Vascular Dementia and combined Alzheimer's-Vascular Dementia are said to make up 80 to 85 percent of all cases of dementia.

The Alzheimer's Association attributes about 8 percent of all dementias to Parkinson's disease although the majority of people who have Parkinson's do not develop dementia. Because of the common symptoms associated with Parkinson's disease such as balance, posture and gait problems, tremors, stiffness and slurred speech, which may make the person afflicted with the disease difficult to understand, his or her remaining cognitive abilities are often unfairly misjudged.

When words fail, there is still touch.

DR. DAVID EISENBERG

Conditions which can cause dementia or mimic dementia include

- brain tumors
- head injuries
- thyroid disorders
- infections such as meningitis, syphilis and AIDS
- alcoholism
- nutritional deficiencies
- depression
- drug reactions

Since some of these conditions are treatable or reversible, diagnosis is, of course, extremely important. In order to diagnose Alzheimer's definitively, a brain biopsy revealing the hallmark plaques and tangles is necessary. However, "physicians can achieve 90 percent accuracy in diagnosing Alzheimer's by performing a thorough evaluation that does not include this invasive procedure."[23]

There is no one diagnostic test that can detect Alzheimer's. A diagnosis is made based on a detailed history, mood assessment, consultation with family members or close friends, and a diagnostic work-up which will usually include most or all of the following:

- a complete physical exam
- CT (computerized tomography) scan or MRI (magnetic resonance imaging) to rule out stroke, tumors or brain changes attributable to other diseases
- neurological exam to evaluate the nervous system, test coordination, muscle tone and strength, and assess sensation
- mental status evaluation to assess person's ability to remember, understand and complete simple calculations
- psychiatric evaluation or neuropsychological testing
- complete blood count and chemistry to detect anemia, infection, diabetes, liver or kidney disorders, thyroid malfunctions or metabolic imbalances
- EEG (electroencephalogram) to detect abnormal brain wave activity[24]

Alzheimer's disease is defined as "a progressive and degenerative disease that attacks the brain"[25] and causes a steady decline in memory, which results in the loss of intellectual functions such as thinking, remembering and reasoning severe enough to interfere with normal daily life. When German physician Alois Alzheimer first described the disease in 1907, it was considered rare. Today, 10 percent of those over age sixty-five and nearly half of those over age eighty-five in America have the disease, which is currently the fourth leading cause of adult death in the United States.

It's Dr. Allan Anderson's weekly visit to the nursing home's special dementia unit, and problems await. Someone hit a nurse. One woman abruptly pinches another patient's face and yells curses. Another breaks into loud, gasping sobs for no apparent reason. Agitation keeps still others awake all night.

LAURA NEERGAARD, ASSOCIATED PRESS ARTICLE

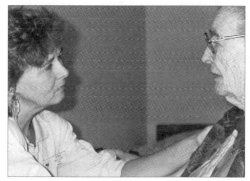

Photographer: Hunter Bahnson

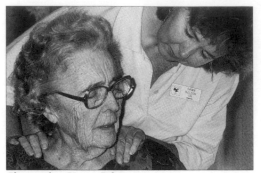

Photographer: Hunter Bahnson

In the Alzheimer's setting, without knowing formal techniques and applications, you can make people feel better just by touching them. If you've had a friend or family member rub your neck for you, you know how good it can feel, even though the person has no formal training.

CYNTHIA BELL, A.C.C.
ALZHEIMER'S DISEASE ED.
CONFERENCE, 1995

A colleague and friend of mine shared her experience of gently stroking a patient's back as he sat with his feet hanging over the side of his hospital bed. Almost immediately, tears spilled down his face, and she heard him say, "Have you ever seen a grown man cry?"

WILLOW DENKER, L.M.T.

HOW TOUCH CAN HELP AS DISEASE PROGRESSES

In the course of its progression, which can last between two and twenty years, with variability in symptoms and rate of decline, this devastating disease gradually steals the mental and physical capacities of those whom it attacks, robbing them of their memory, their independence and their dignity and, eventually, leaving them completely dependent upon others for daily care.

Some advances have been made in recent years and there are now drug treatments that can slow the progress of the disease for some people in the early stages. There is still little treatment available, however, to stop or reverse the mental deterioration of Alzheimer's, a disease which continues to mystify the medical community as both the cause and the cure elude researchers.

Alzheimer's Association literature tells us that approximately 50 percent of nursing home residents and 30 to 40 percent of people in non-nursing home residential care facilities suffer from Alzheimer's or some other form of dementia.[26] More women than men die of the disease, most likely because women generally live longer than men. The number of people living with Alzheimer's disease is expected to increase with the rapid growth of the country's older population. Experts believe that by the year 2050, the number of people with Alzheimer's disease, in the United States alone, could reach 14 million!

A diagnosis of Alzheimer's disease has a significant stress impact, not just the person with the disease but on that person's family and friends. From the moment of diagnosis to the end of life, those afflicted with the disease, along with their loved ones, are subjected to pressures and strains that rarely let up. Compassionate, creative and sensitive caregiving is needed for those living with Alzheimer's disease and for their caregivers, 80 percent of whom report high levels of stress and stress-related illness.[27]

Symptoms that commonly appear in the early stages of Alzheimer's disease can include

- anxiety
- confusion
- short-term memory loss
- mood swings or unpredictable behavior
- difficulty expressing thoughts
- difficulty sleeping
- progressive forgetfulness
- impaired judgment

Skilled touch and massage are beneficial to someone at this stage of the disease, depending on that person's age, in much the same way they might benefit anyone else. Near the onset of the disease, many people are still independently mobile and often able to tolerate a massage session of thirty minutes or even longer on a massage table or sitting in a chair, shifting positions to accommodate the massage. Whatever bodywork techniques or modalities massage practitioners might be using, they should work slowly and sensitively in relating to those with Alzheimer's, with nonjudgmental hands, and emphasizing relaxation.

Those they are working with should be assured that this time is strictly for them, and that there is no need to talk or make any decisions or remember anything important during the massage session. This may well serve to ease the anxiety that forgetfulness and confusion can cause. Nothing should be forced in the session, including the length of time it will continue.

Depression and despair are common side effects for people with Alzheimer's disease who, especially in the early stages, may feel anxious about the future, saddened by what is happening to them and by their awareness of the inevitable progression of their disease. People at this stage of the disease may become emotionally upset or cry easily. Understanding, reinforced by gentle touch, can be a great comfort. Simply being present, listening and receiving whatever is being communicated or expressed, reinforced by attentive touch is also a powerful means of support.

Anger is common, as those newly diagnosed with Alzheimer's or other progressive conditions such as Parkinson's disease are forced to adjust to an altered lifestyle and to a diminishing ability to function in familiar ways. It is important to let these people know that their reactions are normal and that it is okay to express their feelings, whatever they may be.

Each person diagnosed with Alzheimer's disease or some other form of dementia is unique. Although, in the course of the disease, similar terrain may be traversed, there is no certain way to predict exactly what challenges will appear for each individual, when they will appear and how long they may last. It is also impossible to know in advance how severe the challenges will be and how well those affected will adapt. Coping mechanisms and ability to accommodate change vary from person to person. Support systems differ and can affect the impact of the disease for the victims of Alzheimer's as well as their caregivers.

In general, as Alzheimer's disease continues it's assault on the brain, some or all of the following symptoms are likely to appear in what is usually referred to as the intermediate stage:

- short term memory loss
- shortened attention span
- inappropriate responses
- spatial disorientation
- overwhelming confusion
- problems with abstract thinking
- difficulty adapting to new situations
- difficulty performing familiar tasks
- restlessness/"wandering" behavior
- trouble separating fact from fiction
- difficulty listening/understanding

I once met a gentleman at a respite care center who, as he continued to grip my hand after his initial handshake, confided in me that he wasn't sure why he was there and that he found it embarrassing that sometimes he could not remember what he was saying. I assured him that I forgot things too sometimes, and that it was fine by me if we just sat together. I began to rub his back gently with my free hand and told him we didn't have to carry on a conversation, we could just be together in the here and now.

The woman was confused and talking about many different things, wanting to walk in different directions. I redirected her to a chair and gave her a foot massage. Afterwards I saw her walk over to another woman on the unit and look at her feet and try to tell the other person what had just happened. She said words like "good" and "nice" as she looked at her feet.

JUNE KEUSCH, C.M.T.

I have a great feeling for people like my mom needing physical contact... I notice that they all yearn to be touched and they forget so quickly that you have to do it again and again and again. She goes to other respite centers and they have huggers and they are professional huggers... We had a masseuse who used to come to the house, we had a hot tub and she used to come to the house and do massages and mother loved that, we all loved that, she moved away so we don't have her anymore but mother loved that.

DOROTHY JONES, HOME CAREGIVER

Evelyn is a woman who has a lot to say… the language she uses to speak her story is unintelligible most of the time, as far as words go. It appears she doesn't need someone to hear it, for she will sit in the hallway of the facility where she lives and "babble" for long periods of time, as though she just has the inclination to speak. One morning, while I was waiting for a student, I decided to sit down in front of Evelyn and just be with her. She continued to "talk" and, at some point, I put my hand on hers and told her "I wish I knew what you're saying, but I don't." I then began to slowly stroke down her arm from the shoulder, very gently. She seemed to relax into this, so after a little while I did the same thing with her other arm, stopping to spend extra time massaging her hands. For some reason, I felt drawn to put one of my hands on her check, which I did. She closed her eyes at this point, as if she was savoring the touch there. So I put my other hand on her other cheek and just stayed there cradling her face in my hands. A minute or so went by and I realized by the weight of her head and by her breathing, that she had let go enough to fall asleep. She was totally trusting in that moment, and it was my turn to just be there and savor the sweetness of the childlike elder. Eventually, I very slowly released my hands, letting her head drop gently forward so that she could continue in this resting state when I had to leave. Although we seemingly never exchanged an intelligible word that day, I believe that we communicated in a very deep and special way, one that I certainly will never forget. It was a graced morning.

JEANNIE BATTAGIN, C.M.T.

As Alzheimer's disease continues its relentless march forward, symptoms in the advanced stage can include the following mental and physical challenges:

- loss of long-term memories
- regression to childlike behaviors
- inability to communicate with words
- inability to recognize family members
- inability to recognize self in mirror
- little capacity for self care
- hallucinations
- muscle cramping
- incontinence
- limb rigidity
- seizures
- personality changes
- combative or abusive behavior
- weight loss

The person with Alzheimer's disease may eventually be incapable of organizing his or her thoughts enough to carry out even the simplest of activities such as dressing, bathing and even eating.

Women and men in the advanced stages of the disease seem to me to be, quite literally, looking for themselves. They do not know who they are, where they are, what they are or what others want or expect of them. They are unable to demand the dignity and respect they deserve as individuals in our society at the time when they may need it the most.

In the final stages of a progressive illness such as Alzheimer's, so much of the nervous system is failing that the rest of the body is significantly affected. Death may be fostered by a complicating condition such as pneumonia, dehydration or some invasive infection.

Those living with a dementia-related conditions such as Alzheimer's are far from immune to other diseases such as cancer, diabetes, stroke, emphysema, heart disease, and arthritis, nor are they exempt from the gradual decline and physical impairments that generally accompany old age. Coping with any of these conditions can cause added distress and confusion for people with dementia. They may have trouble tolerating prescribed treatments and because people with dementia often have difficulty articulating or explaining their specific symptoms, they may lash out or become agitated instead.

BENEFITS SPECIFIC TO ALZHEIMER'S/DEMENTIA

As previously discussed, the use of massage as a therapeutic modality in caring for those with Alzheimer's disease and other dementias has benefits common to the general population, contributing to

- improved circulation
- pain relief
- stress reduction
- comfort

- calming
- nurturing
- pleasure

The numerous psychosocial benefits of touch therapy sessions for the frail elderly, including those residing in care facilities, may also apply. Such sessions can provide

- skin-to-skin contact
- unconditional one-on-one attention
- companionship
- mental stimulation
- sensory and tactile stimulation
- an opportunity for social interaction
- acceptance and acknowledgment

While little "hard" scientific research is presently being conducted on the benefits of massage for nursing home residents, anecdotal reports from those working in this field have been extremely positive. In a six-month pilot program on using massage therapy as an intervention for problem behaviors in nursing home residents with dementia, conducted at the Methodist Home in Chicago in 1996, a correlation was found between certain kinds of touch, applied on specific parts of the body and specific behavior patterns.

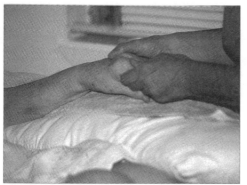

Photographer: Barry Barankin

For example, back rubs worked wonders for those confined to wheelchairs, people in chronic pain and residents exhibiting irritability or even anger. Foot massage proved calming for those exhibiting hyperactive behavior or restlessness and "wandering" behavior. Hand massage or face stroking seemed to help those who were exhibiting anxiety, worry, sadness and fearfulness. Massaging the temples, scalp and forehead helped reduce headaches and tension; and shoulder and neck massage seemed useful for those exhibiting tiredness, irritability or mild upset.[28]

I have found, just as this study did, that rubbing the temples or head is often a strong reminiscence tool for men, just as lotioning the hands can be for women. One man I saw regularly in an Alzheimer's respite care program would say, without fail, every time I gently rubbed his temples toward the end of a neck and shoulder massage, "Well I'd better go jump in the pool now" or something similar. The program director and I eventually surmised that this gentleman associated that particular touch with massages he once received at his country club. Other men may remember a scalp massage as part of a pleasant weekly or monthly ritual in the barber's chair.

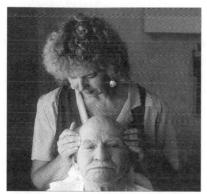

Photographer: Brock Palmer

Alzheimer's disease can erode the mind to the point where the person seems to have no memory at all, no sense of self, and little connection with any physical reality. This can be devastating to loved ones, friends and caregivers, who must watch the person slowly "disappear." When other ways of communicating seem to fail, sometimes the simple gift of consciously focused, caring touch can truly make a difference.

Some years ago, a friend of mine suddenly found herself in the somewhat unsettling position of bringing into her home and caring for her elderly mother-in-law, a woman she had never gotten along with and with whom she had little in common. When I met this tall,

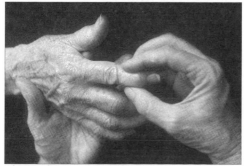

Photographer: James Patrick Dawson

The "massage lady" was sitting near one of our clients who is in the later stages of Alzheimer's when the lady suddenly lashed out at her, and started to hit. The practitioner just took her arm gently and proceeded to move with her, not trying to stop her or force her or anything but just moving with her to the point where the participant got into the moment of gentle exercise and they were doing an arm dance, so to speak. The practitioner stayed with her for awhile and was eventually able to massage the lady's hands and put some lotion on her arms.

JOAN LARSEN,
RESPITE CARE CENTER DIRECTOR

One of our residents is a lady who was quite withdrawn, paranoid, very suspicious of everyone, did not want to be touched. We had difficulty even with the simple daily care activities, like her grooming and hygiene, showering and such. The massage therapist has seen her on a regular basis, has respected her wishes when she doesn't want to be touched, and has worked as far as she can each session with this resident. And we've seen a progression with her, especially in her interactions with other people. She's not as paranoid, not as much of a loner, and she will let people touch her. She will step out of her room into he hallway and I've even seen her walk down the hall to the nurse's station on occasion recently. And I really believe it's a result of the trust relationship that's been built with the massage therapist.

EVELYN YOUNGBERG, D.O.N.

stern-looking woman, her dementia was quite progressed. After being helped out of bed, into her clothes and down the stairs each morning, she spent most of her hours sitting silently in a chair in the corner of the living room doing little more than staring into space. My friend, who knew nothing at all about Alzheimer's disease, grew increasingly exasperated with the woman's behavior and eventually stopped trying to interact with her beyond seeing to her basic needs. Since I was in the home fairly frequently anyway, I asked my friend if I might try offering her mother-in-law some focused touch in the form of massage.

Since I had no history of conflict with this woman, and because I was not the one responsible for the relentless physical care she was beginning to require, I was able to simply be with her and accept her as she was. My friend later made the statement that compassionate touch "reached" her mother-in-law when all else failed.

As a therapeutic tool with benefits specific to Alzheimer's and dementia care, touch therapies can also provide

- a tool for reinforcing verbal communication
- a way of relating nonverbally
- focus for redirecting attention
- a means of distraction if necessary
- a "touchstone" with physical reality

As any dementia progresses, it can greatly limit the activities in which the confused person is able to engage. At some point the person may be unable to remember even the most recent events or to anticipate future ones. Following the action on television or the words of a story tape may become overwhelming. One caregiver told me that although her mother still seemed to enjoy watching certain television programs, she had reached a point where she could no longer use the remote to change the volume or the channel, even when she was holding it. She simply did not know what she was supposed to do with the object in her hand. This same woman responded with obvious and immediate pleasure to one-on-one attention in any form, especially touch. She loved to dance. She loved hugs and back rubs.

Touch is an important tool in relating to those who are no longer able to communicate verbally. Focused touch and gentle massage techniques are often effective as a means of reassuring and calming someone who is confused or afraid. The skillful practitioner can also re-direct the energy when a person tries to communicate by striking or hitting. This type of behavior usually stems from frustration or fear and, indeed, some people in the later stages of dementia seem to be frightened much of the time. Some are easily startled by loud or unusual noises, and some become upset or agitated by any kind of change in routine, by new faces or for seemingly inexplicable reasons. When someone is hitting, the key is not to stop the flow of energy but to channel it in such a way that the person does not hurt him or herself or anyone else.

Touch sessions can help "ground" those who are spatially disoriented and confused by reminding them of their connection with the earth and with other human beings. The actuality of the physical contact provides a "touchstone," so to speak, and a reconnection with something familiar. This reassurance needs to be offered frequently since it is not retained and the memory of the experience can fade in a matter of moments.

Skilled touch has additional benefits in relating to those with dementia in that it can assist in

- increasing body awareness
- focusing attention
- addressing feelings of isolation and abandonment
- engaging attention
- preventing or helping cope with challenging behaviors
- reducing the need for drug intervention

In order to interact successfully with someone living with Alzheimer's disease, you need to feel accepting of and comfortable being with a person who is exhibiting the characteristics of the disease. You must also be able to adapt easily and quickly to whatever situation may present itself. Touch must be offered unconditionally and unobtrusively. It should never be forced or done without expressed or inferred permission (given through observable positive indicators or responses). It is not the particular touch technique utilized that is significant. Rather, it is the ability to be with the person, and to relate to the individual rather than to the disease, the mental state or the behavior, which will build trust and allow real contact to occur.

I think it is good to remember that the individual with Alzheimer's has not always been in his or her present mental state. The person has, in most cases, lived a full and productive life before the onset of the disease, contributing to society and relating successfully to others in many ways. It helps to try to see the wholeness of the person's life, not just what is currently visible.

COMMUNICATION CHALLENGES

Verbal communication problems are often associated with Alzheimer's disease. Trying to understand what those whose brains are affected by Alzheimer's are saying can become a constant struggle. People living with this disease may eventually have great difficulty in making themselves understood at all. They may substitute words, repeat words or invent new words in an effort to communicate. Others resort to a few remembered words to communicate or may even use certain words over and over. Conversely, those with Alzheimer's may be unable to understand what others are saying to them, which presents an equally challenging problem for caregivers.

One of the more bewildering symptoms of Alzheimer's disease, known as *visual agnosi*, occurs when a person retains visual acuity but loses the ability to recognize or correctly identify what is seen. Such perceptual impairments may lead a person with Alzheimer's to misinterpret what he or she sees. The person may become agitated by glare or frightened by objects that he or she cannot accurately interpret.

A more common visual problem in this disease process is impaired depth and spatial perception. Someone facing this particular challenge may have difficulty knowing how much space is between him or herself

> *Our residents have responded to the touch sessions offered on a regular basis in our nursing facility in any number of ways. One that stands out in my mind is a woman with progressed dementia who was unable to communicate verbally. When she was first brought to our facility, she was very agitated and frightened. The massage therapist visited her and she seemed to be calmed a bit by touch. In subsequent sessions, this resident would try to roll up her sleeves and hold out her arms in anticipation of being touched. Eventually, she began to interact with the therapist by reaching out and touching her hands! An even clearer indication of how much these sessions meant to this resident came one day as the therapist was leaving, and the resident said to her in clearly recognizable words, "I love you."*
> BRIANNA ALLEN,
> CARE FACILITY DIRECTOR

We're just sitting here waiting... waiting... waiting...

ALZHEIMER'S UNIT RESIDENT

and another person or object. The author of *Speaking Our Minds*, tells how this particular difficulty affected one of her clients when people offered to shake hands at church:

> "…because of her visual-spatial problems, she was unable to respond: she could not locate the greeter's hand accurately in space… the common misperception was that Bea had become too impaired to recognize the appropriate response to a handshake."[29]

Offering a touch session to those in the advanced stages of a dementia such as Alzheimer's disease can be a real adventure. The most challenging aspect of the work may be getting the person's attention long enough to make physical contact rather than deciding what particular massage technique to use! If you work with someone who has Alzheimer's disease, you must understand that the person may never recognize, remember, or be able to carry on a conversation with you. The person may not want to sit down, or sit still, for more than a few moments, and will never be persuaded through logic or reasoning. Attention spans during the later stage of the disease are very short, and moods may change from moment to moment. Logic and reasoning will have little if any effect in eliciting cooperation. In the middle of a visit or touch session, someone with Alzheimer's may suddenly start giggling uncontrollably, begin swearing loudly, break into song, or simply get up and walk away. Relating to such a person is, in some ways, much like interacting with a small child in an adult body. Communicating effectively with the person or getting him or her to move from one place to another, when necessary, takes a great deal of patience, compassion, understanding and creativity.

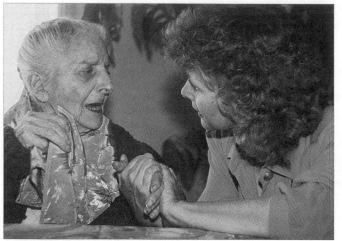

Photographer: Owen Howson

I once had a loquacious client who was no longer able to communicate well through the words she used. She loved music, however, and she loved to move and dance. I was able to use this preoccupation both as a resource for relating to her and as a tool in eliciting her cooperation during our sessions. Staff members in the facility got used to seeing us singing and dancing our way down the hall toward her room. Sometimes we'd stop in the hallway to rest because my dancing partner preferred "the sunshine in the park" (which is how she thought of the well-lit hallway with large green plants positioned every few yards) to the smaller and darker space of her room. Since the wooden bench was exactly like ones that years ago were often seen in parks and gardens, I could sometimes get her to sit by pointing to this piece of furniture and saying, "Shall we sit down on this park bench and have a little chat?" I had to get down in front of her and remove her shoes quickly because she never wanted to sit for long. During her foot massage she would continue humming or chatting in collage fashion about all manner of things.

Although this spirited lady was usually to be found in the designated music room or moving to the music inside her head up and down the hallways, occasionally I would find her inside her room trying to figure out where she was and how to get out. I discovered that I could often get her to lie down on her bed for a back massage by singing to her. In fact, the first time I intuitively began humming a lullaby I remembered from my childhood, she curled up and fell fast asleep!

F is ninety years old and suffers from kidney, bladder, prostrate cancer, Pagets disease and Parkinson's disease. The nurses are amazed at how he responds to me. One time I visited him and was massaging his hands. He took some of the oil off my hand and started massaging my hand… There are times when he holds my hand instead of my holding his. Although most of what he says is not understood by anyone, there are times when we are able to converse a few phrases. This is amazing to the staff.

ROSE GILMOUR,
MASSAGE THERAPIST

Human hearts of all ages yearn for security, affection and acceptance. Age and mental ability make no difference in the desire for basic comforts and human contact. People whose cognitive functioning is affected by dementia-related conditions such as Alzheimer's disease may have lost the ability to communicate in the sophisticated ways that have become familiar to many of us as adults, yet they respond naturally and quickly to music, humor, affection, gentle touch and authentic human contact.

People in progressed and advanced stages of Alzheimer's disease almost always do best relating to one person at a time. They may be easily overwhelmed by a crowd or even by two people trying to relate to them at once. For this reason it is best to minimize potential distractions whenever possible, by shutting a door, for example, or by positioning the person so that he or she is facing a blank wall instead of an open window. However, it is also important not to take the person away from familiar surroundings or to disrupt established routines.

Moods and behavior of the person living with Alzheimer's disease can change frequently and unexpectedly. If such a person seems to be unresponsive or uncooperative, a slightly different approach or simply waiting a few moments before trying the same approach again will often solve the problem.

GUIDELINES FOR SUCCESSFUL COMMUNICATION

Anyone providing care for a person suffering from Alzheimer's disease needs to have a thorough understanding of the symptoms and characteristics of the disease, as well as the ability and the patience to respond to that individual in a compassionate and supportive way. It is important to be very clear and concise in communicating with those who are forgetful, confused or disoriented, without being condescending. Assistance must be offered in such a way that the person suffering from dementia is not demeaned or made to feel incompetent or devalued as a human being.

Successful caregivers and service providers must be continually observant and conscious in learning what works and what doesn't work in communicating with adults living with a dementia-related disease. Some general guidelines for improving effectiveness in interactions with such people are outlined below.

Verbal Communication:

1. Get the person's attention before speaking.
   a. Face the person, making eye contact if possible.
   b. Call the person by name and touch his or her hand.
2. Communicate one idea or one instruction at a time.
3. Speak slowly, calmly and in a normal voice (without raising voice).
4. Use concrete, exact and positive phrasing.
5. Allow the person plenty of time to respond if a response is necessary.
6. Call all people and objects by their proper names.
7. Avoid using slang, nonspecific or abstract words.

K, an eighty-five-year old woman with progressed dementia seemed unresponsive to almost all external stimuli and often sat in a chair for long hours at a stretch, saying nothing and staring into space. Her family caregiver, who knew nothing about Alzheimer's disease, grew increasingly exasperated with K's behavior and eventually stopped trying to interact with her in any way. Doubtful that K would respond but willing to "try anything" she invited me to visit her. The rigidity in K's body began to give way almost immediately when her upper back and shoulders were gently massaged. By our third session, K. was answering direct questions with words instead of nodding or shrugging. Eventually she consented to moving from her chair to the couch so that I could better reach her back and legs to massage them. Although her response to this physical contact may have seemed minimal to an outside observer, I experienced shifts in K's body energy, as well as subtle changes in her demeanor both during and after our sessions.

AUTHOR

We have a gentleman on the Alzheimer's unit that doesn't want to take his shoes off, it just represents something to him that is upsetting. He tends to get very agitated any time someone tries to remove his shoes so giving him a foot massage helped turn this into a positive instead of a negative action. He now associates taking his shoes off with having his feet touched in a warming, pleasurable way.

BRIANNA ALLEN,
CARE FACILITY DIRECTOR

I know of a resident on an Alzheimer's special care unit who frequently complained of someone trying to get in her window at night. Staff members chalked her complaints up to her imagination or perhaps to paranoia or hallucinations associated with her disease, and simply kept assuring her that nobody was there and that she was safe in her room. One evening the administrator of the facility happened to be present when this woman cried out in fright. Upon entering the resident's room, she noticed that a large tree was outlined against the drawn shade by a light shining outside the window. The branches of the tree happened to be shaped in such a way that the shadow did, indeed, look somewhat like a large human figure. Furthermore, a low branch was pushing up against the window so that every time a breeze blew, the branch made a scratching sound against the pane. This resident's fear was easily allayed with a pair of pruning shears.

AUTHOR

8. Minimize arguing or reasoning.
9. Avoid changing the subject abruptly.
10. Give frequent acknowledgment, encouragement and support.

Nonverbal Communication:

1. Make verbal and nonverbal messages the same.
2. Use gestures and facial expressions along with words.
3. Reinforce instructions with gentle physical guidance.
4. Never force physical contact if the person is not open to receiving it.
5. Assume an equal or lower physical position when with the person.
6. If the person seems to become more agitated with physical contact, take your hands away and "hold" the person with your focused attention and presence.
7. Treat the person the way you would want to be treated if you were in a similar circumstance.

Some people who are experiencing the effects of a disease such as Alzheimer's can no longer communicate well verbally, but will respond to key words. Mentioning the key word may jog the memory enough to shift the person's attention and bring him or her a bit more into the present. Making an effort to familiarize yourself with a person's key words and other unique verbal expressions can expedite communication and build rapport.

One resident of a dementia care facility whom I visited once or twice a week referred frequently to "papa," her husband who had been dead for some years. She would become preoccupied with getting home to papa or fixing dinner for papa or wondering where he was. I never felt the need to tell her that papa was no longer alive or that he would be home later. I usually just said "Papa is fine, papa is okay" or "I think papa is resting now." I suppose it could be argued in a philosophical sense, that I could not know with absolute certainty that papa was fine or resting after his death. However, this lady was no longer sophisticated enough in her thinking to engage in such a discussion and I felt certain enough in my terminology to use it. I would then bring this lady's attention to something more immediate by making eye contact with her, showing her some object such as a finger puppet or drawing her attention to the lotion I was putting on her hands.

One day, when I attempted to assist this same lady out of a group room to a more private place for our session that day, she seized the hand of a woman sitting next to her and declared that she could not leave "papa." The woman whose hand had been grabbed seemed less than inclined to play her newly assigned role. I was impressed by the staff member who resolved this conflict before it began by taking "papa's" other hand and leading her out of the room. My client, firmly attached to "papa" naturally followed. I took her other hand and the four of us proceeded down the hallway. When we got to my client's room, the aide led "papa" to the unoccupied bed and sat her down, standing in front of her for a moment. I led my client to her bed and got down in front of her to take off her shoes for her foot massage.

"Papa" got up and promptly left the room, followed by the staff member while my client's attention was momentarily refocused on her feet and our session proceeded without further disruption. Neither the aide nor I ever tried to dissuade my client from her original declaration.

Sometimes, as we were walking down the hall of the facility where this woman lived, she would stop at one of the lovely weavings or original paintings hung in the hallway of her residence and say to me "I made this." I would simply answer that the colors were beautiful or some other positive comment about the artistic excellence and we would continue our walk.

"Little White Lies"

I've seen well-meaning volunteers or caregivers lie to people in advanced stages of a disease such a Alzheimer's, thinking that "they won't know the difference" or "they'll forget the whole thing in a few minutes anyway." In several such instances, I have observed the person being lied to withdraw even further and give up on trying to communicate with that particular person.

Certainly, there are many situations in which fabricating the truth would seem to make things easier or take less time. In fact, I once listened to a whole lecture on how to manage challenging behaviors in people with Alzheimer's in which one of the strategies suggested was telling "little white lies." In a larger context of true relationship, I believe that such a strategy is counterproductive, and that it is almost always better to try to find a way to communicate as accurately as possible, without being cruel.

I will never forget an incident that occurred at a respite care center one day when a regular participant in the program decided that he was going to leave. He went repeatedly to the door and tried to open it. The person in charge kept saying things to him like "Okay you can leave but I just need you to help me do this first" or "Okay you can leave in a minute right after we do this." Such attempts at "redirection" often work because the person soon forgets his or her original intention. However, on this particular day, the gentleman refused to be distracted or dissuaded in his desire. When he was finally told that he could go if he would just eat his lunch first, he hurled his thermos to the floor with such force that it broke with a loud crash, spattering milk everywhere. He pointed his finger at the person in charge and shouted "I know what you are doing and it isn't right" at which point his son was called and asked to come immediately to pick him up and take him home.

I felt intuitively that this man was responding to being manipulated and lied to. If his communication had been acknowledged in some way ("I know you want to go home") and he had been told the truth ("It isn't possible for you to leave right now" or "It isn't safe for you to go out that door alone") and had then been directed to a new activity, I believe he would have responded differently.

Whether a person is two years old or ninety years old, with an immature brain or one weakened by disease, that person deserves to be heard and to have his or her communications, in whatever form they may take, be received and acknowledged.

Toward the end of life, a person with dementia may have only a few words or phrases to stand for all his needs, in the same way that a toddler may say "doggie" for every animal she sees. It's important to know those phrases and their importance to the resident.

KATHY LAURENHUE, M.A.

We have one lady who literally paces all day, up and down the hall. You have to dress her while she walks, you have to get food in her while she walks. When massage was first tried with her, the practitioner literally walked the hall with her, holding her hand and rubbing her back. After about a month of seeing this lady, the practitioner got her to sit down for a good, maybe five, ten minutes, which is a long time for someone who constantly paces. Since then the massage practitioner has taught the aides who care for this lady some simple techniques to use when they're dressing her or during mealtimes. It makes their job easier because this lady is calmer and more relaxed.

BRIANNA ALLEN,
CARE FACILITY DIRECTOR

Occasionally one of the program participants would initially say no to an offer of a back rub so Dawn would just sit with the person, talking about the weather or whatnot, just relate one-on-one and then maybe when she left, they would shake hands or there would be some kind of physical contact. Almost invariably when she returned to that person a little later or on another day, the person would want the back rub. Eventually every single person around the table wanted to be touched and it is wonderful to see how they respond and how much they enjoy this special attention and interaction.

JOAN LARSON, ALZHEIMER'S RESPITE
CARE PROGRAM DIRECTOR

Alzheimer's disease can erode the mind to the point where the person seems to have no memory at all, no sense of self, and little connection with any physical reality. This can be devastating to family and friends, who not only carry the grief of having their relationship to the person go unrecognized but also witness their loved one slowly "disappearing" to the point where that person can no longer recognize him or herself. When a person in this mental state looks into a mirror, he is she may be frightened by the face staring back. In such cases, caregivers usually remove mirrors when possible or try to avoid such potentially upsetting situations.

Several years ago, a student of mine was fortunate enough to be invited to begin offering massage to residents in the multi-level care facility where her training had taken place. The administrator bought a sturdy massage table and cleared out a storage closet and helped transform it into a small but lovely environment where the more active and mobile residents could come to receive massage therapy sessions. She also went into rooms of the less mobile residents to give COMPASSIONATE TOUCH® sessions. This practitioner had one client from the Alzheimer's Unit who liked to walk up to the massage room and get on the special table for her touch session. The first time this lady was escorted to the room and came inside, she noticed an image in the mirror on the back of the closed door and said to the practitioner, "Oh that's my friend. She goes everywhere with me."

A friend of mine told me about a participant in one of her massage workshops who was in the habit of driving some distance each week to a care facility to visit her mother. This woman told my friend that her mother had not recognized her in seventeen years and so she was frequently discouraged during their visits, feeling there was so little she could do to make any difference. After taking my friend's workshop, the daughter tried using some of the basic massage techniques she had learned during her next visit to her mother. Her mother responded to the back massage by smiling at her daughter and saying "I don't know who you are dear but what you are doing feels so good!"

Public awareness of Alzheimer's disease is higher than ever before. Education about Alzheimer's disease is expanding along with community services. Public policies are changing and additional funding for research is available through foundations such as the Reagan Institute, created for the purpose of accelerating the development of effective treatments and prevention for Alzheimer's disease after the ex-president disclosed to the world his own battle with the disease. In the search for new and innovative care strategies for this unique population, massage and touch therapy are emerging as viable modalities for quality of life enhancement and help in managing challenging behaviors.

CAREGIVER STRESS

I know from facilitating caregiver support groups and from observing and talking with those who are full-time caregivers that it can be backbreaking, challenging work, fraught with frustration and difficulties. I have watched husbands and wives give up jobs and activities, use up life savings and sometimes literally sacrifice their own lives to this task. I have seen men and women become sick or physically disabled themselves in the process of caregiving. I have observed the conflict and guilt spouses experience when, for the sake of their own mental and physical health, it becomes necessary to move a loved one into facility care.

The latest statistics from the Alzheimer's Association tell us that one out of ten adults in America now has a relative with Alzheimer's disease. Seventy percent of those with the disease are cared for at home. Eighty percent of Alzheimer's caregivers report experiencing high levels of stress and nearly half of them say they suffer from depression. Long-term unrecognized stress can lead to serious health problems, which is why the Alzheimer's caregiver is sometimes called the hidden victim, or the second victim, of the disease.

Sometimes caregivers are too preoccupied to recognize their own symptoms or need for help or they fail to do anything about them. Stress indicators for caregivers can include

- Unabated feelings of anger toward the person with Alzheimer's
- A tendency to withdraw from friends and family
- An increasing lack of participation in social or recreational activities that once brought pleasure
- Constant apprehension about what the future may hold
- Insomnia caused from worry and anxiety
- Irritability and moodiness
- Exhaustion that makes it difficult to face the day or complete daily tasks
- Depression and despair

It is difficult to continue giving if our own bodies and hearts are not nourished. The wise caregiver will recognize the importance of self-care and will find a way to do what is necessary to preserve his or her own health and sanity. This may involve some creative thinking on the caregiver's part or the ability to ask for help when needed.

One woman who told me that the hardest thing about caring for her husband as his dementia advanced was that he would not leave her side during their waking hours. Shadowing her every move, he grew disturbed if she left the room, and even more distraught if she tried to have someone else sit with him while she ran errands. She said it was easier to send someone else on the errands than to deal with his protracted upset. What she decided to do was get up one hour before her husband every morning so that she could have some time to herself. She felt that getting a little less sleep was well worth it to have some peace and quiet and this seemed to help curb her resentment of her "velcro husband."

Other strategies for reducing stress in caregiving which have been voiced by members of support groups or by caregivers I have known are

Modern medicine is helping us live longer. Today many people in their 70's are caring for parents in their 90's. We are approaching a caregiving crisis in our country.

ROSALYNN CARTER
IN *PARADE* MAGAZINE

- "I go to two support groups and I get a massage once a week."
- "I go to the movies with a friend once a week."
- "I hired a young man to take my mother on drives several hours a week."
- "We hire a caregiver to take mom to a care center one night a month so we can get away by ourselves."

WHAT WE CAN LEARN FROM PEOPLE WITH ALZHEIMER'S

I was given the opportunity, for several years, to spend time each week at a respite center for those with Alzheimer's disease and related disorders. It was usually the most relaxing time of my day. It slowed me down. It brought me into present time. It gave me a chance to practice the art of being truly present, for people in the advancing stages of a disease such as Alzheimer's live mostly in the moment. In this way, they are much like small children. Their emotions are not cleverly hidden, repressed or denied. They are right there on the surface for everyone to see.

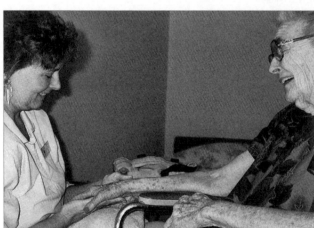

Photographer: Hunter Bahnson

People in a progressed state of a dementia-related disease such as Alzheimer's are in a state, albeit not consciously chosen, that many in our culture spend a lot of time and money and energy trying to duplicate—they live in the present moment! They cannot remember what happened only a few moments before and they give little thought to the future. They can shift very quickly from being frightened or upset to being amused or delighted. At the center, I noticed that almost everyone's face lit up at the sight of a child or a puppy. Most of the participants in the program loved to sing, especially the simple, rhythmic songs of childhood. They laughed easily and responded to honest, real attention.

In my experience, adults with dementia need frequent reminders and respectful guidance just as young children do. And, like children, they are sensitive to dishonesty, subtle manipulation and contact that is inauthentic. They respond positively to genuine contact and gentle, caring touch. Most of all they need understanding, love and support. They are also quick to forgive and they truly do forget.

As Lisa Snyder says in *Speaking our Minds*, "It behooves us as a society to examine our approach to the care of people with Alzheimer's because the extent to which our communities embrace those afflicted is the extent to which we can ensure our own care"[30] should we need it.

For more information on Alzheimer's disease, contact the Alzheimer's Disease and Related Disorders Association, Inc., 919 N. Michigan, Suite 1100 Chicago, IL 60611-1676 Telephone: 1-800 272-3900. Website: www.alz.org

Touch and HIV/AIDS

Receiving a diagnosis of any life-threatening disease is a traumatic event. In the case of HIV/AIDS, the diagnosis is compounded by the unique psychological component of a disease which is known to be transmittable, irreversible and fatal with a progressive course and no known cure. In addition to the sadness, fear and anxiety felt by anyone facing death, those suffering from HIV/AIDS may have internal conflicts and concerns that are seldom issues for people diagnosed with other life-threatening diseases such as cancer. Consider the following:

- Persons diagnosed with HIV are often young.
- Lifelong changes in behavior are immediately required.
- The diagnosis may force a person's identification as a likely member of a stigmatized minority (such as prostitutes, drug users or homosexuals) engendering discrimination and prejudicial treatment.
- The contagious aspect of the disease may cause even close family members to avoid social and physical contact with the infected person.
- The end result of the HIV virus, AIDS, is associated with severe and chronic discomfort, disability and physical disfigurement.
- Fear, lack of knowledge and insensitivity among healthcare workers may be detrimental to care.
- People with HIV/AIDS may be rejected, excluded and ostracized.
- Those HIV/AIDS are vulnerable to feelings of guilt and self-loathing in addition to the fear, anxiety, depression and anger that can accompany any life-threatening illness.

You know somebody with AIDS?
Just touch 'em, man.

CHRISTIAN HERRIN,
FORMER "MALBOROUGH MAN",
HIGH SCHOOL ASSEMBLY TALK, 1994

I once spent time with a young man, barely out of his teens, living with AIDS. He lived in a cluttered but comfortable suburban home that also housed his aunt and uncle and their two small grandchildren. The uncle was diagnosed with cancer during the time period of my relationship with his nephew and they died within a few weeks of one another. I saw this young man every other week, for about six months. He was very thin when I met him and weakened by relentless bouts of diarrhea. His legs were very weak and he spent the majority of his time lying on the couch (his designated bed in the crowded household) in the living room watching television. His interests did not seem to extend much beyond the current soap opera story lines which he would share with me each week as I lotioned and massaged his legs. He spent the last week of his life in the hospital; and when I visited him there, the television was not on. He seemed somewhat troubled and I sensed that he was contemplating his death. After sitting in silence for awhile, holding his hand, I asked him what the hardest thing was for him at that moment. He surprised me by answering "I'm afraid I'm going to go to hell." I was glad I was able to call a chaplain who came to see him the next day and helped him come to some peace on the issue before he died.

AUTHOR

There are also unique psychosocial stresses for those who are in a relationship with the person who is infected, whether they are sexual partners, family members, medical or volunteer caregivers, friends, colleagues, employees or employers. Those people must address their own individual concerns and issues such as

- fear of personal exposure, transmission and infection
- discomfort with an exposed lifestyle
- conflicts with other family members, caregivers, physicians
- the complexity and intensity of physical caregiving and emotional support
- changes in lifestyle and familiar activities
- changes in relationship roles and dynamics
- feelings of vulnerability
- added responsibilities of caregiving and it's physical and emotional toll
- challenges to professional and personal competence
- potential loss and anticipatory grief

TRANSMISSION

If you are involved in caregiving in any way with a person who has tested positive for the HIV virus or who is afflicted with AIDS, you may want to review the following facts in regard to transmission of the virus.

1. The virus needs a specific environment to survive—i.e. blood, semen, vaginal fluids, mother's milk

2. The virus must have a "port of entry"—some way of entering the body

3. A sufficient quantity of the fluid containing the virus must enter the system

The HIV virus is transmitted when the blood or specific bodily fluids of a person who has the virus in his or her body enters the blood stream of a person who does not have the virus. The most common ways for the virus to be transmitted from the body of an infected person to the body of an uninfected person are

- unprotected vaginal, anal or oral sex
- shared needles or syringes

The chances of getting HIV from a blood transfusion in the United States are now extremely low. Babies have been known to become infected in the womb, through vaginal birth and through nursing. The virus has been found to exist in saliva, sweat and tears but not in a virulent enough concentration to cause infection. It was once suspected that some types of mosquitoes might carry the virus from person to person but this has not proven to be true.

Not everyone who tests positive for the Human Immunodeficiency Virus (HIV) and therefore harbors the disease in his or her body will go on to develop AIDS (Acquired Immunodeficiency Syndrome) which is the most harmful outcome of the HIV Virus. Some people carry the virus but remain asymptomatic (without symptoms) for many years, looking and feeling perfectly healthy.

The manifestations of HIV/AIDS vary from person to person and can range from mild to severe. As the virus weakens the immune system, physical symptoms that may develop include

- fatigue, malaise or lack of energy
- headache
- decrease in appetite
- recurrent diarrhea
- weight loss
- recurrent fever
- night sweats
- swollen lymph glands in the neck, underarm or groin area
- white spots or unusual blemishes in the mouth (thrush)

As HIV/AIDS progresses, persons infected with the virus may intermittently experience one or more of the following physical challenges:

- muscle deterioration
- numbness
- rapid aging
- severe joint pain
- neuropathy (nerve damage)
- discoloration in finger and toenails
- gum decay such as gingivitis
- "wasting" syndrome (unexplained continuing weight loss)

The HIV virus can also effect the brain and spinal cord, causing what is known as AIDS-related dementia. Signs of such neurologic impairment might include

- confusion
- difficulty concentrating
- difficulty making decisions
- loss of coordination
- memory loss
- partial paralysis

Opportunistic infections and other complications frequently occur in the advanced stages of HIV/AIDS which can include

- retinitis (causing blurred or decreased vision) and other eye diseases
- respiratory tract and pulmonary infections such as pneumonia or tuberculosis
- malignancies such as Karposi's sarcoma
- bacterial, viral and fungal infections such as tuberculosis, candidiasis, herpes virus, salmonella

Over the course of his or her disease process, the person living with HIV/AIDS is likely to experience a wide range of feelings and emotional responses to his or her diagnosis, disease, treatment and prognosis including

- anger
- anxiety
- denial
- depression

Michael, in his late thirties, was receiving hospice home care after being in the hospital for six weeks. The first day I went to see him, he looked up at me standing in the doorway to his room and said, "Irene, wait, I want to show you something." Unable to walk, he lowered himself from the bed onto the floor. He crawled across the floor to the opposite end of the room and pulled himself onto a sofa. "Watch this," he ordered. Michael took a deep breath through his nose as he brought his hands in front of him, palms out. He opened his eyes and mouth very wide as he exhaled and with the exhale, made large circles with his hands and arms. He repeated this three times. Exhausted, but with a wide-eyed smile, he said, "Isn't that great! That's the first time I've been able to do my yoga in six weeks." Michael then lowered himself from the sofa onto the floor, crawled across the floor and pulled himself up onto his bed. With a gesture of his arm, he declared. "Come on in."
Throughout the next several months of working with Michael, I was deeply moved by his willingness to approach his dying process with passion and creativity.

IRENE SMITH, FOUNDER,
SERVICE THROUGH TOUCH

*I once went to see an articulate
young computer analyst who had
been diagnosed with HIV/AIDS...
He was about to be discharged from
a short term of care in a skilled
nursing facility and, at the time I
met him, showed no outward signs of
ill health. I had been told that
during his stay, he had asked a
healthcare aide for some Kleenex
only to have the woman toss the box
of tissue to him from across the
room! As I applied lotion to his
smooth soft skin, this handsome
African American gentleman
commented on how good the skin on
skin contact felt. He said that he
wasn't touched very often any more
and that when he was touched, it
was always by gloved hands.*

AUTHOR

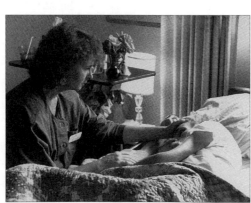

Photographer: Barry Barankin

- fear (of treatment, repercussions, eternal damnation, of death itself)
- guilt (about lifestyle choices, possibility of infecting others, etc.)
- impulsive or erratic behaviors
- mood swings
- panic attacks
- sorrow
- thoughts of suicide

TOUCH BENEFITS

Touch in the form of massage has physical benefits for those with HIV/AIDS common to the general population in terms of

- relieving muscular tension
- lowering blood pressure
- easing stress
- boosting the immune system
- inducing a relaxation response in the body

Massage stimulates circulation in the body, sending more oxygen to the brain. This can temporarily increase mental clarity and counteract disorientation and confusion. Improving circulation in the body can also

- help prevent pressure sores
- combat fatigue
- promote more restful sleep
- increase appetite
- aid in digestion and elimination

The skilled use of touch in caregiving or as a therapeutic modality serves the person living with HIV/AIDS in many other ways that are often more significant than any of the physical benefits already enumerated, due to the unique psychosocial aspects of this particular disease. Compassionate care through intentional touch can

- support the release and expression of feelings
- help raise low selfesteem
- counteract feelings of alienation and isolation
- give comfort and pleasure
- provide a means of nonverbal communication
- help family members re-establish their touch relationship
- increase body awareness
- combat depression
- foster feelings of being accepted and loved
- help produce an experience of wholeness and well-being
- enhance quality of life

Conscious and caring physical contact can fulfill a profound psychological need for someone suffering from a communicable disease such as AIDS. Even with the abundance of information available on how this virus is transmitted, some people remain uneducated or afraid to touch, or even be in close physical proximity with a person who is living with HIV or AIDS.

GUIDELINES FOR TOUCH

If you are relating to someone whose immune system is compromised with a disease such as HIV/AIDS, you must think about protecting that person as well as yourself. If you have not washed your hands, or you have any kind of open lesion, contagious rash, cold or infection you are putting them at risk. A scratch, hangnail or infected skin area on the end of a finger can be covered by a finger cot. (Boxes of latex finger cots can be purchased in drug stores. Each box contains several sizes so that you can find the right one that will fit snugly wherever you need it.)

Here are some other important guidelines for touch practitioners and caregivers to observe when providing massage or hands-on comfort care in any form to someone with HIV/AIDS.

1. Wash your hands thoroughly before and after your touch sessions with an antimicrobicidal soap and warm water.

2. Remember that your intact skin is a protective barrier.

3. Healthcare professionals who work in medical and extended care facilities are required by law to wear gloves when touching (for any reason and in any way) the body of someone diagnosed with a communicable disease such as HIV/AIDS. As a volunteer caregiver or touch therapist, you have the freedom to make your own decision as to whether or not to wear gloves when you are coming into physical contact with someone living with such a diagnosis. It is, however, important to use disposable latex gloves if

    • you will be coming into direct contact with blood, urine, feces, semen or vomitis
    • you have any cuts, scratches, contagious rashes or open lesions on your hands
    • there is any chance you are putting the person you are touching at risk of infection
    • the person you are going to touch requests that you wear gloves
    • you feel uncomfortable touching the person without wearing gloves

4. Scan the body of the person you are going to touch for weeping lesions, open wounds, rashes, fungi or any condition that might require special attention or which you need to avoid touching.

5. Learn the difference in contagious and non-contagious rashes. Herpes, for example, which is a common infection in people with HIV/AIDS where it may be especially prolonged and severe, is contagious to caregivers and can be carried from one part of the affected person's body to another part.

6. Ask questions if you are in doubt.

7. Seek the support of others who are working with those who have HIV/AIDS to share your experiences, express your feelings and to raise issues of concern.

TAKING CARE OF YOURSELF

"Having an HIV client pierces the shield that protects us from life and death issues."[31] We must recognize the emotional impact of working with the seriously ill and learn to be self-observant, so that we can make sure our own needs are met, and so that we can grow from the experience. In conjunction with suggestions given elsewhere in this book in regard to self-care and dealing with loss and grief, here are some additional strategies for handling the intensity of the questions that arise and the issues that emerge around death and dying.

1. Know your limitations.

2. Be willing to set boundaries.

3. Watch for signs of stress, overwhelm or burnout.

4. Develop strategies for meeting your own physical, emotional, psychological and spiritual needs.

5. Allow time for processing loss and grief.

For a free copy of the year-end HIV/AIDS Surveillance Report call the CDC National AIDS Clearing House (1- 800-458-5231)

For a copy of "Guidelines for Massaging HIV Infected Persons," and a list of other resource materials and workshops available, contact Irene Smith, 41 Carl St., #C, San Francisco, CA 94117

The Power of Touch in Caring for Our Dying

As "baby boomers" age and our parents grow even older, and with AIDS, cancer and heart disease reaching epidemic proportions, it is hard to avoid death any longer. Many of us are caring for dying loved ones or grieving their deaths and beginning to come face to face with our own mortality.

Receiving a diagnosis of a life-threatening illness, (or being closely related to someone who has received such a diagnosis) is listed close to the top of any list of stress-producing situations. The person who has been told that he or she has an incurable disease is faced not only with the immediate sense of loss of control but with myriad anxieties, fears and concerns. "How much time do I have left?" is often the first thought, followed by questions about what course of treatment to follow, what the effects of the disease as well as treatment for the disease may be on mobility, lifestyle and quality of life and so on. Many people worry about how to convey the news to family and friends, about the cost and potential burden of their care, about the ability of surviving family members to take care of themselves and about how, where and with whom to spend the rest of their lives. The decision-making process can be exhausting, especially in combination with recovery from surgical procedures or other types of treatment and with the emotional impact of a "terminal" diagnosis.

...people who are very sick long to be touched...

SOGYLA RINPOCHE

A colleague and friend of mine, Helen Campbell, was once asked to see a woman had just received a devastating medical diagnosis. The woman had been crying for hours and apparently neither the hospital chaplain nor the social worker had been able to calm or comfort her. Helen didn't try to talk this woman out of her grief. What she did was show the grieving woman's husband how to give his wife a simple back massage. After a few minutes, as he continued rubbing his wife's back, the man made some offhand humorous remark. His wife laughed and the mood of despair was finally broken.

AUTHOR

The family of a gentleman in a nursing facility asked me to visit him for massage. He had Parkinson's disease and during our early sessions, he used a motorized scooter and loved to meet me in "the parlor" as he called it. He was very responsive to the massages and we became friends. As he physically declined, he no longer could use the scooter and it became difficult for him to speak or eat. It seemed that he was approaching death and his family asked me to increase my contact with him. His son told me that the massage was the "only remaining pleasure he has". As he weakened and seemed near death, I changed my approach and would sit with him, simply touching the areas that he previously liked to have massaged. He appeared very fearful and seemed to be clinging to life. As I spent time with him in his final days, I experienced an acceleration of my own inner growth. This friend taught me something about life through his death, and I thank him.

ANN CATLIN, L.M.T.

I was all alone when the doctor told me. It was just like in the movies. The first thought I had and the first question I asked was "How long do I have?"

FRAN GUERRERO, CANCER PATIENT

Nurses and other caregivers have observed that patients' need for pain medication is often reduced after massage or touch sessions. I believe the reduction in pain after such sessions can occur for a variety of reasons. It may be because the tactile stimulation has improved circulation in a particular area, allowing energy to flow more freely. It may be that the one-on-one attention and nurturing the patient has experienced through his or her contact with another has allowed him to relax and soften to the point of becoming more accepting of his pain. It may be that the person being touched feels acknowledged because someone else has understood his or her predicament or discomfort and has paid attention! Whatever the trigger that induces the relaxation response, the person who is relaxed often finds her or his condition less stressful and more tolerable.

We all know what pleasure memories can bring. Receiving a massage can evoke pleasant memories of earlier times of being touched, and the memory itself can trigger a relaxation response as well as bring enjoyment. My services were once requested for a hospitalized cancer patient who was experiencing a great deal of discomfort, particularly in her arms and shoulders. She was eager for massage. She was experiencing so much pain on the day of my first visit, however, that even the softest touch on her upper arm or shoulder proved to be too much. A large tumor growing in the upper node of one lung was pressing on a nerve, and apparently responsible for the shooting pains down her arm as well as the burning sensation she felt in her fingers. This spirited forty-two-year-old woman was very much awake and aware even though she was taking medication, including morphine, for her physical pain. Her condition reminded me of a woman's labor pains before birth, as the intense discomfort came upon her intermittently and demanded all her attention. She apparently noticed the similarity too, commenting wryly that dying of cancer was harder than giving birth.

I asked this feisty woman if she would like a foot massage, to which she gave a resounding "Yes, I'd love that!" As I moved to the end of the bed and began massaging her feet and legs, her husband, who was standing nearby, mentioned to me that his wife could no longer feel anything below the waist! I continued what I was doing, knowing that even though she couldn't feel my hands on her skin, the massage would help the circulation in her legs. What I didn't realize, until she told me, was that she enjoyed watching me massage her feet and legs because it helped her remember the pleasure that she and her husband had experienced in giving each other foot massages. She could also experience a slight sensation in her upper body when I held her feet and gently pulled. She even joked that I was "pulling her leg!"

COMMUNICATING WITH THE DYING

When you are working with someone with a very serious or "terminal" illness, you may be able to sense when the end is very near and you may not. Death, like birth, comes in its own time and can sometimes occurs when we least expect it to. I have known people who appear to be on the brink of death, yet they linger on the precipice for many weeks or even months. I have known others who, though seemingly stable, caught everyone unaware and suddenly slipped out of their bodies.

The point is, that although the awareness may be heightened when you are in a relationship with someone who has been declared near death, in any relationship every time you say good-bye, there is a chance that you will not see that person again. It is desirable, therefore, to keep communications current.

I worked with a particular gentleman in a hospice program over a period of seven months, weekly in the beginning and eventually twice a week. I had grown to cherish this person and always looked forward to our visits. One day, as I was leaving, I spontaneously kissed Bob on the cheek and from then on it became an important ritual of our parting each time we were together. As my friendship with this man, and my affection for him and his wife grew over the months, I had the impulse several times to say "I love you" to him, but for some reason I just never did it.

As I was getting into my car to drive to Bob and Mary's home one morning, I noticed a particular rose blooming in the garden and had the thought that he might like it. I then reasoned that if I took the time to go back into the house to find the clippers and a container to put the rose in to keep it fresh for the thirty-minute drive, I might be late for our appointment. I decided I would wait and take one of the roses to him on my next visit two days later.

When I arrived at Bob's bedside, he seemed in a slightly weaker condition and less talkative than usual. There had, however, been many ups and downs in the course of his disease and so I really didn't think too much of it. Looking back on it, I remember being reluctant to leave at the end of our session but as I told him goodbye that Tuesday morning, I said I'd see him on Thursday. After his death the next morning, I regretted not having taken him the rose. And, even though I know he knew it, I regretted never having told this unique individual that I loved him.

It is best to avoid the "I'll see you next week" type of goodbye when taking leave of someone who is nearing the end of life. It is better to say something like "I'm glad to have seen you today" or "It's been good

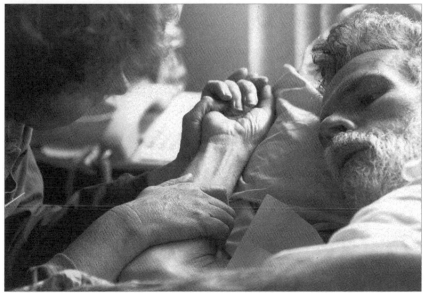

Photographer: Barry Barankin

I was caught in a big snow storm in Victoria, British Columbia, Canada. I was visiting friends who lived next door to a hospital for the elderly. The hospital had called asking for help in feeding the patients. Four of us went for the next three meals. At the evening meal, I was asked to feed the women in room ten. The first bed was occupied by a beautiful, white-haired woman, Ann, who couldn't speak but responded well as I fed her. I was very conscious of the second woman in the room, Jean, who was too ill to eat.

Jean was a very small woman, very sick and her arms were up from her lap and trembling. Quite spontaneously, I turned from giving a spoonful of food to Ann, to stroke Jean's forehead. Her head was quite cool, but as I went from a spoonful of food for Ann, to stroking Jean's head, she seemed to like being touched and so I continued going from one person to the other. At one point, I realized that her hands were resting on her lap and no longer trembling. I had to go to other patients. I stood at the foot of Jean's bed and told her I had to go. She opened her eyes and looked at me. I will never forget the expression of gratitude in her eyes. I walked up to her again, kissed her on the forehead and left. Hours later, she died.

I had never seen this person before. Why I was there that night when they were so short of help, I'll never know. I may have been the last person to touch her. What a privilege to have been with her!

SARAH COMEAU

I had fallen into an easy camaraderie with F. and his wife during my weekly visits to their simple, comfortable home. F.'s wife was always warm and welcoming. She often sat in the room reading or sewing as I gave F. a foot massage, which we hoped would help stave off the threat of pressure sores. He enjoyed having his hands massaged as well. His wife seemed to have adjusted well to her role as her husband's primary caregiver and, with some help from the hospice team and from their adult children, a routine had been established that was working well. F.'s medical condition seemed stabilized. I perceived little change over the few weeks I was privileged to spend time with this lovely couple. I always ended my time with F. with a lingering handshake; and he and I usually exchanged smiles and a moment of silent contact before I left. On this particular afternoon, as I held F.'s hand and bent down to adjust his pillow before leaving, he winked at me and whispered "This is it." He died peacefully in his sleep that night.

AUTHOR

to spend time with you." It frees the person mentally and emotionally to engage in the task of dying, whenever the task presents itself, without encumberment.

I have known several people, including my father, who held on to life until a loved one was able to "let go" or become more accepting of the impending reality of death. I have known of people who died within hours or minutes after being released in this way. Some caregivers are appreciative of a gentle suggestion in this regard; others are not ready to let go and will not be receptive to such an idea. If a caregiver or loved one of a person near death expresses a thought about how long a death is taking, it creates an opening to introduce the idea of communicating his or her acceptance of the death directly to the person. I have sometimes accomplished this through sharing a story about someone else's experience in this regard.

As the physical body continues to weaken, a person near death may begin to detach or de-identify with his or her physical existence. That person may start communicating in symbolic language, in regressed language, or without the use of words. We must make room in our minds and hearts for the dying person's experience, whatever it may be, staying open to communications offered, in whatever form they may take.

Often people approaching death will give some kind of clue to indicate that they feel the time is near, or as a way of telling you goodbye. It may be something very simple or subtle, something which could be easily overlooked in a different situation.

One woman whom I had visited over a period of several weeks was in a great deal of pain and spoke very little during our last session together. She was resting in a hospital bed that had been placed in the living room of her home. I remember that she was experiencing severe headaches as well as confusion and anxiety. When it was time for me to leave, she seemed reluctant to let go of my hand and held it tightly for some minutes. I knew that she had a fear of dying alone. I was able to tell her that she had many people who cared about her (neighbors, church friends and relatives, along with her healthcare team, had arranged a schedule so that someone was always there) and that whatever happened as things progressed, she would not be alone. I also assured her that we were all committed to helping her to be as comfortable as possible.

As I opened the front door to leave that day, I turned back to look at this sweet and fragile lady who had essentially remained curled up under her blankets and facing the wall since my arrival. She turned her body toward me and raised herself slightly from the bed, looked directly at me for the first time that day. Then she said in a relatively strong and clear voice, "Goodbye Dawn. Have a good evening with your family." I told her I would be thinking about her. I'm sure she sensed, as I did, that we would not meet again. I was not surprised to receive a phone call less than two days later telling me she had died.

When a person nearing death speaks of wanting to go home or wondering where home is, family members often assume that the person is confused or delirious, overmedicated or that the disease the loved one is dying from has affected his or her brain. I have been greeted at the door by more than one anxious caregiver who has been understandably upset over this apparent loss of logic or the dying person's inability to communicate clearly. One distraught mother who had been single-handedly caring for her adult son for many months told me tearfully "I keep telling him he is home. This is his home." Some diseases can cause dementia as they progress, yet it is also common for a person nearing death to speak of home or of wanting to go home, as a way of indicating a desire to leave the body. Someone may speak of needing a passport or a plane ticket, or wanting to get to the bus stop as a way of saying that he or she is ready to make a change or to go on to a new or different place. I remember my father, who had always enjoyed watching sports events such as football and basketball, speaking to me over the telephone a week or two before he died about trying to get to the end of the football field. He told me he could see the lights on the other side of the field but that he just couldn't seem to get to them.

As our loved ones, friends or clients approach death, we can support their journey toward this moment of transition; and we can share in their experience as long as possible by accepting rather than resisting, refuting or denying what is being said. We can let them know that we are open to listening and receiving anything that they want to share, and that it is all "okay."

Gayle MacDonald writes in *Medicine Hands* that:

> *Touch for the dying should also be freeing, allowing them to be unfettered, rather than binding them to this plane…our hands and our hearts must be open, not clutching; they must be light, still and calm, asking nothing, offering thanks and release. We must create an*

> *I was bathing a patient and her mother was holding her and she died in her mother's arms. Her mother said 'I held her as a baby when she came into the world and I'm holding her now as she leaves the world.' It was wonderful to witness that.*
>
> DOROTHY CHAKNOVA,
> HOSPICE HOME HEALTH AIDE

J and his wife were cultured and gracious people. Their exquisitely decorated apartment was filled with art objects and relics from their world travels. Ballroom dancing had been a passion and a pastime for them since J's retirement. He greatly enjoyed having his legs and feet massaged once a week. After his session, I would often give his wife a short back rub or a foot massage as we all sat and visited in their living room or den. J was a large man and his wife rather petite. As his physical needs became greater, she found it more and more difficult to cope with caring for him. They made a decision together for him to go into a nursing home to be cared for there. Shortly before his death, I visited J in the nursing home. When I arrived J seemed to be napping and a woman I had not seen before was sitting in a chair in one corner of the room, looking quite nervous. She was an old family friend. When I encouraged her to come sit on the other side of the bed, she silently mouthed the words, "I don't know what to do." A few seconds later she came over and gave J a quick kiss on his forehead and then hastily left the room just as he opened his eyes and said "So sweet to have known you." Although he smiled in recognition when he saw me, I was sorry that his words had missed their intended recipient. A few minutes later J said to me, "I don't want to miss a minute of this." I understood that he knew he was beginning the dying process and that he wished to stay conscious as long as possible. Over the next two hours, as I sat with J, several extraordinary things occurred. At one point, summoning strength from some unknown place, he unexpectedly and with great determination climbed over the rail of his bed and stood up, saying his son was coming to pick him up and that he had to go to him. I told him that I would walk with him. I was concerned that he might fall and wondered if I should call for help when he quickly forgot about his mission and his strength ebbed… I helped him get resettled comfortably in his bed, lowering the rail so I could get my chair as close as possible to the bed. I sat with him in silence for some time, holding his hand. I thought he was asleep when, without opening his eyes, he tapped his forehead with one finger. I asked if he was experiencing pain and he said softly, "No, tightly confined." At another point he sat suddenly upright again, putting his legs over the edge of the bed. He seemed remarkably awake and alert, his eyes wide open, a kind of innocent wonder on his face. He put his hand to his heart, tapping gently on his chest and then said in a lucid, clear voice, "There is so much love, I never knew there was so much love." As far as I know those were the last words J spoke. He soon fell into a deep sleep and I went home to my family. When I came back the next day he was still sleeping and died a few hours later.

AUTHOR

I had for several months been visiting a young woman who had contracted HIV from a companion of seven years who told her he'd never had sex with anyone else. By the time I met her, the companion was dead and her own death was not far off. Her body was already thin and wasted and she was no longer able to walk. She lay in a hospital bed in her widowed mother's double-wide trailer home. One morning when I called to confirm my arrival time that day, I could hear the anxiety in her mother's voice as she asked if I could come any sooner, saying that her daughter seemed to be "slipping away." When I arrived, her daughter was awake and coherent and she did seem to be intently focused on her dying process. I encouraged this young woman's mother to sit where she could maintain eye contact, as well as physical contact, with her daughter. I stayed on the other side of the bed where I could stroke her back. Time seemed to suspend in a sacred space as I witnessed the two women tell each other goodbye. The mother, with tears streaming down her face, was eventually able to tell her daughter that she was releasing her and that she should just leave her body and float toward the light. The daughter told her mother how much she loved her and that she would miss her. After some time had passed, she curled up, almost in a fetal position, and began speaking in shortened phrases and a child-like voice. She would drift off and then open her eyes again, find her mother's face, and repeat, "I go bye-bye now... I go bye-bye." This continued throughout the day until she fell into a coma a few hours before her death.

AUTHOR

emotional spaciousness within ourselves that allows the dying person the freedom to be on any plane necessary...[32]

I have observed people who know they are nearing death regress in their use of language, and begin using words that they may have used when they were very young or first learning to speak. This seems to be especially true in cases where an adult child is being cared for by a parent.

It is possible that all speech will stop as the body weakens. Words may eventually seem superfluous, yet the person approaching death will continue to communicate with those nearby through touch, gestures and facial expressions—a smile, a wink, lips pursed in a kiss, a hand squeeze or a little wave. I have observed loved ones who are able to set aside all else and be present at such a precious time stay in intimate communion with the dying person and carry on very loving "conversations" in this way.

It is also fairly common for those who are transitioning into death to suddenly smile and reach out, or seem to be visually focused on someone or some thing that no one else in the room can see. Research has proven that in the near death state, people often see loved ones who have already died, angels, lights, images of religious figures or other indescribably beautiful visions. Some people hear beautiful music or simply sense the presence of their beloved nearby. I have observed this phenomenon several times.

Rather than feel excluded when the person seems to become aware of something that we are not experiencing, we can support the person by staying consciously present and in contact with him or her. There are many stories of people near death who report seeing angels, other dieties or loved ones who have already died in their room or standing beside them. It is not uncommon for those near death to report seeing a bright and beautiful light just ahead.

There are no rules. There is nothing to "do." There is no right or wrong way to die or to companion someone who is dying. We can honor the individual and the sacredness of the transition by simply surrendering to the contact that unfolds within the context of our relationship with another, trusting that appropriate touch or other ways of lending support will present themselves in the flux and flow of the moment. You cannot change the script of an individual's life nor can you prevent death, but you may be able to help someone die with a measure of dignity, supported by human contact.

People are often thrilled to be invited to help in or bear witness to a birthday process. People are less frequently invited to attend a death and even those who are may have qualms about going. "Deathing" is not viewed with the same celebratory and anticipatory thoughts as "birthing", yet both transitional events can be awesome and sacred experiences. Being present to that holy moment of a life completing itself and moving out of the body can transform as well as inform our lives.

Death can be a tumultuous time, precipitating turmoil, trauma and sorrow. It can also be a time of peace and healing. Death offers the opportunity for communion and communication that can deepen and renew our sense of connection with others.

THE BENEFITS OF TOUCH IN HOSPICE CARE

In medieval times the word *hospice* referred to a way station where travelers could be refreshed and cared for. Today hospice is a program of care that attempts to provide for the physical, emotional, psychological and spiritual needs of those who are approaching death. In recent years, public interest has engendered open discussion about death and about more compassionate treatment of those diagnosed as "terminally ill." Hospice has become a strong force in the search for a more unified and holistic approach to life and death, emphasizing more humane and compassionate care for the dying.

The basic purpose of hospice is to enhance quality of life, regardless of the expected duration of that life. In hospice care, the primary goal is to help individuals coping with diseases considered to be incurable to live as fully and comfortably as possible, in familiar surroundings and in the company of family and friends.

A requirement for acceptance into most hospice programs in America is that the person applying must have received a diagnosis from a medical professional that his or her disease is likely to lead to death in six months or less. If death has not occurred in that length of time then the person's situation is reassessed for current status and need to be in the program. I have known a few people who have "graduated" from hospice when a medical condition stabilized or even improved. Hospice promotes the right of patients with a life-threatening illness to be heard, to be told all the facts, to share in decision-making, to refuse treatment, to try "alternative" treatments, to maintain as much control over their own lives as possible. It also ensures the right of persons in the program to be cared for by professionals and volunteers who have respect for them and for their families.

Some hospice programs are community based, relying on grants and community or donated funding for their existence; some are privately funded; and others are part of medical centers. In some cases, hospice care is provided in a specific location or a designated residential unit. Most modern American hospice programs, however, offer care to patients in their own homes.

The majority of hospice patients have some form of primary cancer that has metastasized (spread) to other parts of the body. Other hospice patients suffer from respiratory conditions, cardiac disease, neuromuscular conditions such as Parkinson's or ALS (Lou Gehrig's disease), and some have AIDS.

With an emphasis on caring for the whole person, hospice programs often provide many benefits that are not available in traditional health-care settings. Specially trained volunteers are an integral part of patient care, providing companionship, respite for caregivers, and social and emotional support to patients and families.

In addition to on-call nursing, spiritual counseling, bereavement support and psychosocial services, patient benefits may also include music, art and massage therapy. These "alternative" therapies are sometimes included in allocated budgets and sometimes payment to the providers comes from donated funds. Massage support to family caregivers may or may not be included in these models. In other hospice programs, massage and other services considered to be

After his massage sessions, my husband has a reduced amount of pain for the rest of the day and is able to sleep for several hours without medication.

MARY LOVEJOY,
WIFE OF HOSPICE PATIENT

The hospice team was invaluable. Without hospice she would never have had the quality of life that she did.

MOTHER AFTER DAUGHTER'S DEATH

A patient I was seeing weekly, after the fourth or fifth week was able to go on reduced medication for pain relief.

DEANNA MATTHEWS,
C.M.T., HOSPICE

complimentary to medical care are only available if someone in the volunteer pool can offer them.

Relating to the seriously ill and the dying through the medium of massage has numerous benefits for both the receiver and the giver. Skilled touch in the form of massage has many of the same physical benefits for hospice patients that it has for anyone else in that it can

- soften contracted or tight muscles
- relieve tension in the body
- promote faster healing from injury or trauma
- improve joint stiffness
- calm the nervous system
- reduces anxiety
- induces overall relaxation response
- boost the immune system

Massage and touch therapy offer additional support to the seriously ill and the dying by

- helping in pressure sore prevention and healing
- providing a means of nonverbal communication for those no longer able to speak
- providing non-pharmalogical pain relief
- helping reduce the need for sleep-inducing medications
- helping maintain body awareness
- providing reassurance that the patient is not alone
- helping to sustain feelings of self-esteem and self-worth
- helping calm the spirit as well as the body
- encouraging emotional expression
- acknowledging the continued wholeness of the individual
- helping reduce feelings of isolation and loneliness.

For some hospice patients, the psychosocial benefits of touch are significant. People confronting a life-threatening illness usually experience a kaleidoscope of emotions in their process of coming to terms with their approaching death, such as

- **anger** about the diagnosis, physical and mental limitations imposed by the disease or effects of treatment
- **anxiety** about treatment pain, finances, how family members will cope
- **denial** about the diagnosis or the progression of the disease
- **fear** about what will happen next and about death itself
- **guilt** over how the situation is affecting loved ones
- **mood swings** caused by the stress, drug therapy or disease-related dementia
- **depression** and **hopelessness**
- **thoughts of suicide**

The right touch at the right moment can be far more effective than words in acknowledging a person's suffering and offering comfort and support. Conscious, attentive touch supports an individual in releasing feelings and active listening encourages the person to express those emotions.

A MODEL FOR MASSAGE IN HOSPICE

The hospice program I was associated with for five years, first as a volunteer, and then as a massage therapist on independent contract, was part of a large, nationwide Health Maintenance Organisation (HMO). Home-based hospice services were available to any HMO member and covered a fairly wide geographical area. Patients in the six-bed in-patient unit in the hospital for emergency procedures and respite care were also included in all services offered. The hospice team at that time also included a music therapist and an art therapist, all paid from donated funds. As more and more requests for massage sessions were received, more therapists were brought in. By the end of my association with this particular hospice, there were four therapists working with about ten different patients at a time, more than a third of the total census. Each massage therapist was paid a flat fee regardless of length of the visit or mileage incurred. Massage support to family caregivers was offered, if requested as part of the home or hospital visit.

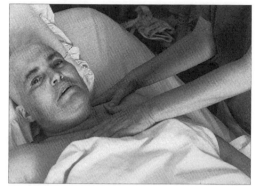

Photographer: Michael Pederson

Each person admitted to the hospice program was given a packet of materials that included information about the massage therapy program, which was available to all participants in the hospice program at no extra charge to the family. The service was offered on a priority basis according to assessed need and availability of a practitioner. Each session was individualized, with special consideration given to the unique situation and needs of the hospice patient. The length of the massage session was geared to the individual's desire and tolerance for touch.

A massage therapy referral form was available to all team members. Information on this form included

- patient's diagnosis
- reason for referral
- assessed need (low, medium or high priority)
- who originated the request
- reason for request (i.e. muscle spasms, relaxation, stress management)

A massage therapist was occasionally requested for a one-time home visit, to teach some simple techniques to a caregiver or to help calm a family member who was particularly overwhelmed or distressed. More often, however, once the referral was made and the massage practitioner made contact with the patient and his or her family, visits were continued on a weekly or bi-monthly basis until the patient died. Follow-up visits for bereavement support were allowed if the caregiver had already been receiving touch from the practitioner.

A record of each session, including responses, observations and recommendations, was completed by the massage practitioner after

*You must communicate with each
other and with the person you are
taking care of. You have to be open,
you have to communicate whether
you want to or not. You have to face
reality whether you want to or not,
no matter how painful it is. It
doesn't make it any less painful but
it makes it bearable.*

MOTHER OF HOSPICE PATIENT

each session with a patient or his or her caregiver. That form was then filed in the patient's record where it could referenced by other team members. Any specific problems or questions that arose during a session were immediately telephoned in to the patient care coordinator, or the appropriate member of the hospice team for attention. The primary care nurse could be alerted, for instance for areas at risk for a pressure sores. Dry or itching skin could be reported to the home health aide so that a different soap or after-bath lotion could be used during the next visit. If a caregiver seemed particularly overwhelmed or under stress, the social worker assigned to that case or the volunteer coordinator could be notified so that extra help could be sought or respite care recommended.

Weekly team meetings were held for the purpose of disseminating information on families new to the program, reporting on recent deaths and covering special interest topics. The meetings also provided an opportunity for brainstorming with the entire team in regard to specific concerns or challenges. Bereavement support and grief processing for team members was offered bi-monthly in the form of group meetings with a psychologist

GUIDELINES AND SUGGESTIONS

In caring for the ill and the dying, you will encounter situations that simply do not occur in other contexts. You may need to hold a container while someone vomits or you may be called upon to help change a foul smelling diaper. It may be necessary to aspirate a mouth full of saliva in the middle of your session or to stop whatever you are doing and just hold someone while that person screams or cries. You may be tempted to run out of the room or to scream or cry yourself. You may be the only person present when someone takes her or his last breath. You cannot deny or repress your feelings. Nonetheless, you must learn to notice your reactions and to put them aside (to be examined or processed later) in order to be fully present with the person/s you are choosing to support.

Remember that you are touching a person as soon as you enter the space that she or he occupies. You are touching with your energy, with your attitudes, with the quality of your presence. People who are seriously ill are often extremely vulnerable and sensitive to touch, to sound, even to the thoughts of those around them. Remember also that you are touching more than a physical body as you make contact with your hands. If your energy is consciously focused and you are attentive to the individual, then you are touching heart and spirit as well.

Anyone who touches traumatized and weakened bodies must, of course, use common sense in avoiding direct contact with open sores, wounds, bandages or bruises.

Avoid any pressure on or rubbing across duralgesic patches (these contain medication that enters the body through contact with the skin). It is possible to gently massage around such areas or to do energy work just off the body, directly above them. It is important, of course, to take appropriate precautions when touching people who have infectious diseases such as Hepatitis B, HIV/AIDS, or with a person who is suspected to have tuberculosis.

Touch is a powerful catalyst in releasing emotions. Someone in a fragile and vulnerable state may respond to attention through touch by relaxing enough to release emotions that have been held in check or to talk about something he or she has been unable to discuss with family members. At other times, your touch may allow a person to sink more deeply into silence or enter into a meditative state. In general, massage sessions with hospice patients will be shorter in duration than those with other clients. The situation may change frequently and what worked or felt good to the patient one day will be inappropriate or intolerable on the next visit.

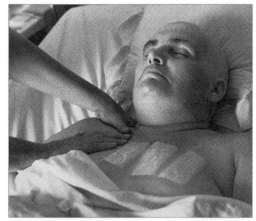

Flexibility and creativity are essential in working with those nearing death. Problem-solving sometimes requires seemingly unorthodox solutions. I remember visiting one man who was resting in some discomfort in the middle of a king-size bed. He was unable to move and I was unable to reach him from either side. The caregiver had taken a break and the man really wanted his back rubbed. So I crawled up on top of the bed quilt as gracefully as possible and gave him a back massage.

Photographer: Michael Pedersen

I have also given mobile massages. I remember one rather eccentric lady who was simply not comfortable sitting or lying down, and felt better when she kept moving. Rather than try to persuade her to lie down so I could massage her, I held her hand and walked with her, giving her a back rub as we moved. Eventually she decided to try lying down on her bed and was able to relax and be nourished by receiving some gentle massage for almost twenty minutes. When you are working with people who are experiencing less and less control over their lives, it becomes important to let them make as many decisions as possible.

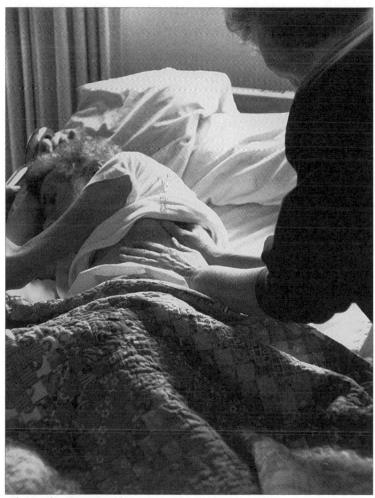

Some seriously ill people sometimes feel more comfortable, initially, with a loved one or caregiver staying in the room during a touch session and that should certainly be allowed. It may reassure that person and reinforce the legitimacy of what you are doing. It may also help the caregiver or loved one feel more comfortable about using touch as part of his or her caregiving.

I was once working with a cancer patient who was very close to death. The day I arrived for what turned out to be my last session with this woman. Her sister, who happened to be visiting, asked if she could stay in the room and observe what I was doing. I was happy for her to do so. After her sister's death, I received a note from this woman telling me that being present for the massage session had given her the confidence to touch and stroke her loved one in the short time they had left together. She said that her experience really taught her how important touch was in such a situation.

Photographer: Barry Barankin

*They said you were angry and
they were right of course.
Yet beneath the anger
was a scared little boy,
crying out for his mother
to make this bad thing go away,
longing for a father who could
somehow accept him,
lonely for the brothers he felt
had betrayed him,
grieving for the friends
who had already died.*

*I found you grasping
at the edge of bitterness
for a piece of understanding,
waging war against a monster illness
and the demons of your mind.
When your mother came at last,
love swallowing her terror,
to spend three weeks with you,
you gave her two days only
for the seven years she'd missed,
before you cast aside your wasted
    body
and moved beyond our sight.*

AUTHOR

EMOTIONAL IMPACT OF WORKING WITH THE DYING

In relating to the seriously ill and the dying you will encounter unique circumstances and a wide variety of situations. Many of the people you see may be experiencing intense personal turmoil. Some may still be in shock from receiving a diagnosis of an incurable illness, or traumatized by the effects of surgery or treatment such as chemotherapy, radiation and other medical procedures. Some will be traumatized, confused, angry, overwhelmed or in despair. The person facing his or her death, and all those who love that person, will be in various stages of denial or acceptance in regard to the death; and each one may have different reactions and coping strategies.

You will have no control over the environments you encounter. The ambience in the home of a person nearing death can range from chaotic to serene.

There may be extra people and auxiliary equipment in the home, which can add to a feeling of confusion and disorder. You may be trying to relate to the dying person in the middle of a space fraught with tension.

It takes a good deal of emotional stability to keep your equilibrium and perspective if you are spending a lot of time with people in the midst of the intensity and turmoil that often surrounds death and dying. It requires paying attention to your own behavior patterns and watching for signals of stress or imbalance.

Some people who work on a continuing basis with individuals nearing the end of life and in the active process of dying report that the work becomes almost addictive. I think one reason this occurs is that being in the presence of people who are approaching death galvanizes our attention in a way that everyday life may not. It awakens us to what is actually important and real; and it keeps us focused in present time.

Another reason why spending time with the dying may have such great appeal is that we have a deep desire to unravel the great mystery of human experience that we call death. We have so much to learn about how to approach death and so many questions about how to do it. Sitting in quiet contact with a person nearing the completion of a lifetime, being in the presence of someone who is about to withdraw from a dysfunctional body, witnessing the transitional moment when an individual moves from one realm of existence into another brings us a little closer to participating in and resolving that mystery. In this way, spending time with the dying can be exhilarating and even liberating.

In working with the dying we are given the opportunity to expand our ideas of what death is, of what help is, of what healing is. I have witnessed miraculous healing take place within individuals and within families as death approaches—healing in the sense of acceptance, wholeness and completion.

Caring for the dying offers us a chance to know people we would otherwise never meet and to share in some of the most precious and sacred moments of their lives. It offers the possibility of looking more deeply into our own fears about death and dying and into our resistances to meeting life as it is. It affords the opportunity to feel both the strength and the fragility of life, and to experience a deeper gratitude for each moment as it unfolds.

Being physically present with those who are near death gives us a unique opportunity to confront our own mortality. It helps us examine our resistances to life and our resistances to death. It gives us a chance to face our fears about living and about dying. Seeing someone ill and in pain reminds us that we could be that way too. It brings up thoughts of how it might be if and when we receive a "terminal" diagnosis. Will I be disfigured? Will I suffer horrible pain? Will I lose control of my bodily functions? Will I lose my hair or my eyesight or my ability to speak? Will I be a burden on my family? Will I become mentally incapacitated? Watching someone die makes us think of how we felt or how we may feel when someone we love dies. It makes us wonder what it will be like when we die. It helps us confront our attachments and our helplessness; and it gives us the chance to greet our own pain and grief with mercy.

Relating to the dying can be challenging, uncomfortable, emotionally draining, fatiguing and even frightening. It can also be peaceful, inspiring and enlightening. It evokes our deepest grief. It inspires our highest thoughts. It takes us to the edge of what we know and pushes us into new awareness. The opportunity for growth is enormous. In caring for the dying, we are called upon to let our hearts break, to let go again and again, to leave our egos behind, to stay present in the midst of our sorrow and our fear and to surrender to the actuality of life and death.

As caregivers and companions, sitting in the presence of a person who is actively experiencing the transition from what we call life into what we call death, we are changed. If we allow ourselves to open to the experience, those who are dying, as Rachel Naomi Remen says "…give a sort of darshan to the rest of us in the same way spiritual teachers do."[33]

FOR FURTHER INFORMATION ON HOSPICE:

Contact the National Hospice Organization, 1901 N. Moore Drive, Suite 901, Arlington, VA 22209, 703-684-7722 to identify hospice programs in your area.

All hospice volunteers are required to complete a thirty-two-hour training, which also functions as a screening process. In addition to learning how various members of the hospice team contribute to patient care, trainees have the opportunity to explore their own feelings and share their experiences in regard to death, dying and bereavement.

I happened to be visiting in his home when my brother-in-law was diagnosed with cancer. While there, I gave him a touch session, using a particular bodywork technique I was trained in. It was the beginning of his interest in complimentary medicine and a strong bond between us. Although we lived on opposite coasts, we stayed in close contact over the three years of his illness. He continued to have bodywork done and felt it was of great benefit.
When the call came telling me that Tom was close to death, I felt I had to be there. When I arrived, Tom was actively dying, struggling to breath and agitated at times. I told Sandra I could do a simple technique that might help him relax enough to let go. She wasn't ready then but early the next morning she came and got me out of bed. Tom's brothers and wife surrounded his bed as I touched him. He began to relax, his breathing calmed and within minutes he was gone. I could feel the peace in his body as left it; and I felt fortunate to be able to say good-bye to him in this gentle, heartfelt way.

TERRY FEIGENBAUM

SIGNS OF APPROACHING DEATH AND APPROPRIATE RESPONSES

1. Body extremities become cool to the touch and may turn slightly bluish in color as blood circulation slows down. Person may complain of feeling cold.

    Use any gentle touch techniques you feel are appropriate or that the person requests. Work on top of covers or reach underneath to administer massage if necessary to keep the person warm.

2. Increase in time spent sleeping and some difficulty in arousal from sleep due to changing body metabolism.

    Assume that the person can still hear everything that is being said and may still experience pain. Use attentive touch techniques. Sit quietly with the person, putting your attention on the individual. Practice the shared breathing meditation described in the chapter on Complimentary Relaxation Techniques.

3. Disorientation and difficulty identifying people, time or place, also due to changing body metabolism.

    Remain a calm and reassuring presence. Give physical and verbal contact. Tell the person who you are, where he or she is and who else is nearby.

4. Decreased need for food and liquid intake as body naturally weakens and begins to conserve energy.

    Refrain from "pushing" the person to eat or drink. Respond to any requests that are made. Accept the way things are. Provide intentional, caring and very gentle touch.

5. Incontinence (inability to control urine and/or bowel function). Urine may darken and amount passed may decrease as kidneys begin to shut down.

    Help with hygiene as needed. Give verbal and physical reassurance and support. Remain focused, calm and present.

6. Restlessness, random hand movement, hallucinations, visions which may be due, in part, to decrease in oxygen circulation to the brain and changing body metabolism.

    Accept whatever the person says, hears or does. Remember that acknowledgment is not necessarily agreement. Maintain physical contact. Give verbal reassurance of your presence. Remain open to the individual.

7. Irregular breathing pattern with ten to thirty seconds of no breathing as circulation slows down and body waste products build up.

    Breathe with the person. Maintain physical and eye contact if possible. Remain attentive and open to each moment as it unfolds.

8. Saliva pools at back of throat, due to decrease in liquid intake, increasing weakness and inability to cough up or swallow normal saliva production. Condition may produce noisy, congested or gurgling sound sometimes called "death rattle."

Try turning the person gently onto his or her side, using pillows to give support behind the back and putting something under the cheek to catch secretions. Or put a pillow under the person's head to elevate it slightly. A cool mist humidifier in the room may be helpful. Stay present and in contact with the individual.

These are some of the conditions or states you may observe in a person who is within a few days, hours or minutes of death. They may not all occur. It is possible that none of them will occur.

PHYSICAL CHANGES WHICH OCCUR DURING AND AFTER DEATH

1. Signs that death has occurred may include

    *   cessation of breath
    *   no movement
    *   no detectable heartbeat or pulse
    *   no response to verbal or physical contact
    *   eyelids slightly open and eyes fixed on one spot
    *   relaxed jaw, leaving mouth slightly open
    *   involuntary loss of bladder and/or bowel control

2. Rigor mortis (muscular rigidity) begins two to four hours after death. This contraction of muscle fibers that immobilizes the joints begins first in involuntary muscles, heart, GI (gastro-intestinal) tract, bladder and arteries. It proceeds to the voluntary muscles of the head and neck and then to the trunk and lower extremities. Rigor proceeds until full intensity about forty-eight hours after death.

3. Algor mortis, or cooling of the body, this is the second noticeable change after death. After circulation closes down, bodily fluids stop their movement and begin to settle. Internal body temperature begins to fall at approximately one degree per hour. Body temperature continues to drop until it approximates room temperature, which is why the skin feels cold to the touch.

4. Decomposition. The third major change which occurs after circulation in the body ceases is the beginning of decomposition, which manifests as a softening of the tissues and discoloration, making the skin appear mottled or bruised or both.

Qualities Worth Cultivating

Specialized training in massage or specific forms of bodywork may be useful, especially for those wishing to earn a living as touch practitioner working with the elderly or the ill. It is, however, not necessary to be a professionally certified or licensed massage therapist in order to offer compassionate care through touch. Regardless of our roles in life, we all have the potential to grow in our sensitivity and our compassion in relating to others and to develop confidence and competence in the art of communicating through touch. Almost any human being has the potential to use touch as a form of hands-on healing. Inherent abilities can be expanded and specific skills learned which can be integrated into any caregiving situation to enhance quality of life for the elderly, the ill and the dying.

Some people are naturally adept in the artistry of "reaching out and touching" others through the spoken or written word. Other people seem to possess a natural tendency to communicate through their touch. They just seem to have a special facility for tactile contact. Such people often become known for the gentleness of their hands, the nourishing fullness of their hugs or for their ability to offer just the right touch at just the right moment. Their touch makes a difference.

There are other qualities or characteristics that seem to support favorable relating to the elderly and the ill through the use of skilled touch. Some of the attributes I have observed in those who are the most successful in using touch in a conscious, caring way to enrich their caregiving or to help enhance quality of life for those in facility and hospice settings are outlined below.

The hands of those I meet are dumbly eloquent to me. There are those whose hands have sunbeams in them so that their grasp warms my heart.

HELEN KELLER

It is well known in professional circles that young nursing students tend to avoid touching elderly patients...

ASHLEY MONTAGU

ADAPTABILITY

In teaching workshops around the country, I have found that highly trained massage professionals sometimes have difficulty adapting their skills to being with the elderly and the ill, many of whom may be wheelchair or bed bound, in a weakened or confused state, unable to effectively communicate their needs and, in some cases, unable to tolerate more than a few minutes of focused touch. Relating to the frail elderly and the infirm is quite different from practicing massage in a spa, sports or studio setting with able-bodied men and women who are comfortable for an hour or more on a massage table and who can tolerate deeper forms of bodywork.

Most massage professionals are used to being in control of the environment in which they work. They have explicit goals in their work and are used to effecting a change in their clients through the practice of particular massage or bodywork techniques. They are also used to getting verbal feedback and direction from the person they are massaging.

I often tell such students that in our work it is probably best for them to forget much of what they've learned in massage school—forget about the word "massage," forget about the various bodywork techniques they may have spent a lot of time, money and effort in perfecting and go back to the very basic concepts of touch and contact. I tell them it may behoove them to let go of their techniques and their goals and their agendas in favor of simply being present with another human being, putting their attention on that person as an individual and letting the relationship, which may or may not include physical contact, unfold. Some of them don't listen or ignore what I'm saying and then when they go on the Alzheimer's unit or visit the dying on the third day of the workshop they begin to understand. At that point they usually feel a "call" to spend more time with fellow human beings in such circumstances or I never hear from them again!

The ability to adjust quickly to a variety of circumstances in different environments is essential for the caregiver or touch practitioner who hopes to work with those in later life stages. Care facilities come in a variety of shapes, sizes and styles. They can vary vastly in terms of types of populations, how they are run and their governing policies. Staff turnover rates are often high and, just as a presidential election can change a nation, different administrators may have completely opposing agendas and styles.

The volunteer or touch therapist visiting hospital patients or care facility residents has no control over the overall environment and little over the space occupied by the person he or she is seeing. Sights, sounds and scents in the environment are constantly changing. There may be numerous interruptions and distractions. Some people will be unable to speak or to move. Some will be confused, disoriented and uncooperative. Some may get up and walk away in the middle of the visit or touch session.

Caregivers must be able to adjust quickly and easily both to the environment and to the changing physical, psychological and mental states of the people they are caring for. When relating to the frail elderly and the seriously ill, everything from the caregiving team to the medications being taken is apt to change and shift with some frequency. Life can be very unpredictable in the healthcare facility. It is important to be able to adapt to different surroundings and to become comfortable in a variety of situations.

The person who is unable or unwilling to adjust and adapt to constantly changing, new and unfamiliar conditions will soon be exhausted by his or her resistance and will lose interest in relating to others under such circumstances.

TOUCH SENSITIVITY

I once had a student who had already graduated from massage school when she took a three-day training workshop from me. She later attended several one-day seminars I gave and also scheduled a private consultation for the purpose of obtaining advice on marketing her massage skills in care facilities. However, for some reason, no matter how hard she tried, she seemed unable to create the kind of touch practice she desired.

A year or two later this woman called to ask if she could return a video she had purchased from me, saying she wasn't going to be pursuing her dream of offering massage to the elderly and the ill any longer. In the course of our conversation she told me that she did not have the ability to feel through her hands how a person was responding to her touch. She expressed regret that she had gone all the way through a massage school program and none of her teachers had discovered this. I was somewhat chagrined to realize that I had not noticed such a significant point either.

Dr. John Upledger, creator of CranioSacral Therapy, a gentle hands-on method of evaluating and enhancing the function of the craniosacral system, once said that his best students were middle-aged women who had finished raising their children. He said these women had a natural familiarity with physical contact as a means of communication, many of them were already skilled at observing and understanding subtle signs and indicators in the physical body. In addition they were practiced at using touch to comfort, to nurture and to heal.

Physical contact is not the same as caring touch.

EVELYN YOUNGBERG, D.O.N.

An ability to feel the response of another and to sense the effects of your touch is a critical attribute when you are making a physical connection with another human being for the purpose of supporting healing. Without such sensitivity, it is difficult for a touch relationship to grow or to affect either person.

Your hands feel like music on my skin.

ELDERLY CLIENT
TO JUNE KEUSCH, C.M.T.

INTUITION

When you simply understand or know a thing without going through any intellectual or logical process to come to that understanding, you are using an internal system of perception known as your intuition. To be intuitive means to be able to perceive or become aware of something through a source other than the thinking mind or the senses. This intuitive ability might be referred to as listening to your inner voice, listening with your heart or sensing what is best, as opposed to thinking too much about what to do or coming to a logical decision.

During one of my last visits with a woman in her forties whose cancer had spread throughout her body, she kept pointing to a nearby wall and asking her husband to close the door. He ignored the request at first and finally, somewhat annoyed and confused, told his wife that there was no door where she was pointing. Finally, raising her voice, she said "Well just humor me and shut the (expletive) door will you?" Her husband walked over to the wall and banged his hand against it, saying "Okay, it's shut" and then walked out of the room. I suspected the request was her way of saying that she wasn't ready to die. My hunch was confirmed when she turned to me after her husband left and said, "I'm not ready to go through that door yet!" I asked her what she needed to do before she'd be ready and then told her I was pretty certain that whenever she was ready, the door would open again for her.

AUTHOR

The ability to access and use your own inner wisdom is of great value in life. Intuition becomes particularly important in relating to the seriously ill or to those near death who can no longer communicate verbally, when relating to someone with dementia who is unable to communicate reasonably or when relating to someone who speaks a different language than the one you speak.

Working intuitively and in contact with each individual, you will eventually know what part of the body to touch as well as when and how to touch it. You will know when to listen and when to speak. You will act appropriately and accurately in most situations. Cultivating a connection with "the teacher within," and learning to follow this inner guidance gives you access to a valuable reservoir of information that can be of great help in relating to those in later life stages.

An intuitive leap may occur when the mind is confronted with something that it cannot easily grasp or assimilate. In this sense, working with those who are critically, chronically or seriously ill, dying or disabled gives you the opportunity to become more conversant with your intuitive nature. It is your intuition, as well as compassion, which will allow you to sense the innermost thoughts, fears and needs of another. As your heart opens to what your mind may not easily absorb, you will rely more on your intuitive wisdom to reveal to you what to say or not to say, how to touch, where to touch and when not to touch as each moment unfolds.

ABILITY TO FOCUS

The ability to keep your attention and your energies directed toward one person or one thing at a time is a valuable skill to possess in any endeavor. In fact, it is very difficult to accomplish anything without focus!

In touch or massage sessions, there are two important areas of focus. One is keeping your attention on the person you are touching. To do this, you must develop the ability to notice when you are distracted as well as the ability to set aside any distractions that draw your attention away from person you are there to serve. Distractions could be anything from your own mental thoughts about the person's physical condition to a housekeeper running a vacuum cleaner in the hallway. One distraction comes from within your own mind and the other from the environment.

Random, casual touch does not have the same effect on either the person initiating the touch or on the recipient as touch that is offered in a focused, conscious and mindful way. When touch is perfunctory or purely functional and task oriented, it does not promote connection or relationship. In fact, being touched repeatedly in a mechanical, habitual, aimless way can generate feelings of disconnection and even annoyance.

It is easy for your own thoughts and feelings to splinter your attention in subtle and almost imperceptible ways. You may be the kind of person who can think about or do several things at the same time and so you find you are planning what to prepare for a family dinner while you are giving a foot massage to an elderly patient in her hospital bed. Although it looks the same to an observer, this experience is not the same for the person you are touching or for you, as the experience of keeping your attention focused completely and only on that other person. You can experience the difference for yourself by doing the following exercise with a friend or loved one:

> *Sit down with the person you have chosen to do this exercise with. Let yourself get comfortable. Take a deep breath. Look at your partner. Put your attention on him or her for a moment. Now take one of your partner's hands between your own two hands. As you hold your friend's hand, begin to apply a gentle squeezing pressure. You do not have to look into the eyes of your friend while doing this. Do keep your attention solely on her or him. Now, purposely and consciously continue holding and massaging your partner's hand and think about something else. In other words, take your mental attention away from what you are doing and from the person you are touching and think about someone or something else, or look around the room or out the window until some object catches your attention. Just let your thoughts wander where they will. Now, ask your friend to tell you what he or she experienced. Switch roles so that you can experience being the recipient of touch that is, at first, focused in a conscious, attentive way and then given in an offhand, casual and random way.*

You may experience a dramatic change when the attention of the person massaging you shifts away from being totally focused on you, or you may only notice a subtle difference the first time you try this exercise. Ask your friend to tell you what it was like for him or her to touch you with focused attention and then with divided attention.

Another kind of focus that is beneficial in the context of touching others is the ability to direct your energy in a physical way. In other words, you want to be able to channel or to allow the life force or life energy to flow out of your body and through your hands to reach and connect with another. Practice the following exercise when you want to remind yourself of the reality of this energy or when you wish to refocus your attention on experiencing the energy that emanates out from your physical body:

> *Sit upright in a chair. Be comfortable and, at the same time, make sure your spine is straight (that you are not "slouching" down in the chair). Inhale and exhale slowly and deeply. Take a few moments to notice your relationship to the ground beneath you and to feel centered inside yourself. Now, bring your open hands together in front of your body with the palms facing each other a few inches apart. Keep breathing normally and focus your attention on the palms of your hands. Begin to very slowly move your hands a little closer to each other and then a little further apart, noticing what occurs or what feelings you experience as you do this.*

The heart that breaks open can contain the whole universe.

JOANNA ROGERS MACY

*Put down your opinion, your
condition, your situation, then you
will not be stuck. Always stay open.*

SEUNG SAHN

*Practice moving your hands even further apart and notice at
what point you feel a change in the sensation or connection
you feel between your two hands.*

*(Note: if you are having trouble experiencing any changes as
you do this exercise, bring the palms of your hands together
for a moment, rub them back and forth vigorously a few
times. Notice the heat you are generating. Now try the
exercise again.)*

*You can do a similar exercise with a friend, putting your two
open hands in front of you with the palms facing the palms of
the other person. Experiment with focusing your attention on
experiencing the energy field that builds up between your sets
of hands as you move them closer and farther apart.*

When you put your attention on your own life force or energy, you
may experience it as a tingling sensation or perhaps as something like
an electrical current moving through your body, or even as heat or
light or pulsation. You may experience the energy flowing inside or just
outside your body. Once you have focused your attention on this
energy and experienced it, you can experiment with consciously
directing it. As you breathe from your center, you can practice letting
the energy move from that place up and into your arms, down into your
hands and out through your fingers.

As you concentrate on focusing and directing your energy, you will
notice that this skill eventually becomes automatic. You may feel it
more intensely at times or moving through you in different ways; yet
you will no longer have to think about it each time you begin to touch
someone.

ABILITY TO ACCEPT THE WAY THINGS ARE

It is essential to develop the ability to stay consciously present from
moment to moment, whatever occurs. If you can let go of your desire
for things to be different and accept the way things are, your responses
and actions are more likely to be appropriate to each individual and to
each situation as it unfolds.

You may well encounter people who are physically connected to all
kinds of medical equipment and apparatus. You may be relating to
people who will be exhibiting varying degrees of alertness and
coherence of thought as well as varying degrees of physical and
psychological pain. You may be relating to people whose physical and
mental condition changes drastically from day to day, even from hour
to hour. It is quite possible to be touching a person in her or his last
hour or minute of life.

The people you see may be connected to various kinds of medical
apparatus and devices such as oxygen tanks, catheters, feeding or IV
tubes and monitoring equipment. You may need to work around
narcotic patches, diapers, bandages and so on. The person you are
caring for may be confused and disoriented from the effects of drugs,
emotional trauma, overwhelming anxiety or disease-related dementia.

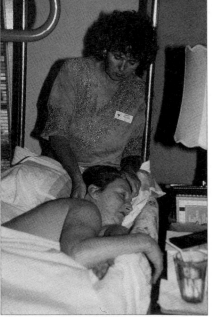

Photographer: Barry Barankin

There is an element of unpredictability any time you are interacting with human beings in crisis. Offering support and relief to those who are nearing death, challenges you to remain flexible and adaptable. It challenges you to accept things the way they actually are rather than the way you may wish they could be.

OPENHEARTEDNESS

To enter into an authentic relationship with another, we must be open and receptive. In relating to the frail elderly, the ill and the dying, the heart must expand to include that which we might rather not see or feel. We must open to that which may be new and different and even frightening to the mind; and we must learn to "see" with our hearts.

The challenging aspect to opening your heart to another is that doing so leaves you vulnerable and unprotected in a certain sense. You cannot really open to another without also being open to your own feelings of sadness, fear, loneliness and anger. Choosing to be open brings you closer to those whom you want to serve and, at the same time, opens the door into your own subconscious. Your openness will bring your own fears into the light of consciousness and perhaps into expression, so that they have less power over your mind.

Your open-heartedness will infuse your caregiving with greater reality and will add dimension to your touch sessions. Opening your heart to the individual you are caring for, being with that person just as he or she actually is, and surrendering your ego in service to that individual can significantly affect your life.

SENSE OF SELF

Being well grounded in the reality of your own being is an important quality to develop. In other words, it is beneficial to others for you to have a conscious awareness of your own physical presence, and a clear sense of your physical and psychological boundaries.

One reason this sense of self is important is that without it you may find that you begin identifying with the people you are touching or taking care of to the point of "merging" with them emotionally, mentally or energetically. While this is an interesting metaphysical exercise, it is not, ultimately, the best way to serve others in the context of caregiving.

If you are not a person who always feels naturally "grounded," or physically connected to the earth, it may be helpful for you to practice bringing your attention and awareness to your physical being. I use the following exercise to remind myself of the simple fact that I am in a physical body walking on the earth and supported by it. (It is also a good technique to employ when you "fly off the handle" and need to regain your composure.)

> Close your eyes and bring your attention inside your physical body. Inhale deeply through both of your nostrils and then exhale through your mouth. As you exhale, feel the density of your physical body as you sit or stand on solid ground.

As my workshop participants dispersed to various rooms for their practice touch sessions with the facility residents that Sunday afternoon, I noticed a staff person walking authoritatively up and down the halls with an air of confidence and purpose, although she did not seem to be engaged in any particular task. What was interesting to me was that her attention seemed to stay above the heads of the residents she was passing. She never acknowledged their existence, never touched or spoke directly to any of them. It was as if they were invisible to her. Her demeanor was in sharp contrast to that of another staff member who was also moving up and down the halls that day. This woman put her attention briefly on each person she passed, smiling at other staff members, stopping to hug a resident or to kneel down beside a wheel chair to make eye contact, touch someone's hand or tuck in a lap quilt. The difference in the two attitudes was truly remarkable. It seemed to me as if the first woman's heart was closed and the other woman's heart was open. Her presence warmed the space while the first woman's presence chilled it.

AUTHOR

Become conscious of the reality of your body in contact with the solid matter beneath your feet. Experience the floor or ground in contact with your feet and, by extension, feel the earth supporting your physical presence on it. To carry this grounding exercise further, you might imagine an invisible but impermeable pole extending from deep within the center of the earth, coming up through the surface of the ground and into your body. Imagine this pole continuing upward through the center of your body and emerging from the top of your head, extending up into infinity. Continue breathing, remaining consciously aware of your body supported by the earth and upheld between earth and sky.

Another aid in experiencing a sense of self is the ability to remain centered, or in touch with your own inner energy source. Here is a simple centering exercise, which you can do either sitting or lying down.

Close your eyes and let your body relax. Let your belly soften. Now breathe deeply into your belly. Take another full, deep breath. Find the place inside your own body that feels like the center of your physical being. Just notice where that seems to be for you. It may be near your navel or lower in your body or it might even be around the area of your heart. Continue your abdominal breathing and keep your awareness inside your own body until you feel completely calm and centered within. If your attention wanders, bring it back by focusing on your breathing as you inhale and exhale... You may want to imagine a bright light or an energy source originating in the center of your physical being and radiating outward through all parts of your body, including your hands and fingertips.

ABILITY TO PUT ATTENTION ON THE INDIVIDUAL

The ability to put your attention on another person as an individual is one of the most useful skills you can develop in relating to those who are ill, elderly or near death. This ability will, in fact, help you greatly in all your relationships. When I speak of the individual, I am referring to something other than someone's physical appearance, personality or behavior. I am talking about something that does not change, regardless of an aging process, a disease process, a deformity or a disability. It is something other than the body, the mind, the ego, emotions, thoughts, feelings, perceptions, awareness and all the other things that we identify as being who we are.

With practice you can develop your capacity to see beyond a disabled, disfigured, decaying body, to see beyond a cranky or argumentative personality. You can develop the ability to keep your attention on the individual rather than on an agitated mind or on a painful physical condition. With practice you can begin to de-identify the individual not only from his or her body but from states of being or from particular points of view which are being expressed. It is useful to notice that points of view, mental states, emotional states and physical states all change. Yet the individual exists and is there throughout the changes which the body or the mind goes through.

Noticing a person's state of mind and the physical condition of the body that person inhabits, especially when you are about to touch the body, is important. If, however, your attention stays focused only on a person's suffering, physical condition or anxieties, you will be less able to serve that individual. You will be trying to contact that person through your reactive mind rather than from a centered, focused and balanced state of consciousness.

I am not suggesting that you should be blind to or unaffected by the pain or suffering of someone with whom you intend to work. I am saying that the most compassionate thing and the most conscious thing you can do is to notice your reaction to the person's condition and then put your thoughts aside in order to be present with the individual who is in that condition or state.

I once volunteered to massage a man who had been suffering for nearly fifteen years from a rare neuromuscular disorder. This particular disease causes severe involuntary muscular contractions in the body, usually in the shoulders, the neck and the face. In this person's case, the right shoulder was in continuous spasm and the head was being pulled to one side by constant and irregular jerking movements in the neck. As a result of this constant movement, the man's jaw had been pulled out of alignment. This affected his speech and made it difficult to decipher what he was saying. The progression of the disease had eventually made swallowing so difficult that his entire diet was in liquid form and given to him through a gastrostomy tube, as were all his medications. He used a machine, much like those that dentists use, to aspirate saliva when it collected in his mouth. He had developed the habit of holding a small handkerchief over his face and mouth or between his lips. This was partially to hide his face from visitors, perhaps to alleviate their discomfort as well as his own, and partially to keep his teeth from biting into his lips. The spasms were more or less violent from day to day and he sometimes had a continuous tick near one eye which gave him the feeling that there was some small object in the eye causing incessant irritation. His urine was passed through a catheter and collected in a bag hooked to the side of his bed. An oxygen tank and mask, as well as an IV stand, stood ready beside his bed.

Needless to say, I had never met anyone with this particular disease or in this type of ongoing predicament before. I was somewhat overwhelmed with the sight that greeted me as I walked to this gentlemen's bedside. A number of thoughts and feelings arose in me as I began touching him. I felt great sadness for him and for his wife. I felt fear that I, or somebody I loved, could suddenly be afflicted with a disease such as this person suffered from. I wondered how I would cope with such a tragedy. I felt a bit guilty that this man had been in this helpless physical state for so many years while I was healthy and actively walking around. I was filled with a desire to "help" this person, to "do" something to alleviate his pain and suffering.

93

Whatever there is of God and goodness in the universe it must work itself out and express itself through us.

ALBERT EINSTEIN

Everybody has had a mother and a father and sooner or later we've got to treat our elderly clients the way we would our own parents.

WORKSHOP PARTICIPANT

Instead of taking a moment to notice and acknowledge my reactions to the situation and then give my attention to the gentleman who was bedridden and disabled by this unusual disease, I tried to ignore my emotions, override everything I was thinking, and administer massage therapy. I wasn't centered and I wasn't really relating to this man as an individual; I was in a mental daze and simply "going through the motions." Consequently, I came away from my first visit with this man somewhat numb and, eventually, in physical and emotional discomfort myself. If he had died before our next session, I would never have known him. I would have remembered only a body in pain, rather than the miraculously pleasant, loving and gracious man who inhabited that body. It was a dramatic lesson for me, and one that I have never forgotten.

The following poem, addressed to her nurses, which I first saw quoted in a newsletter from Lagunda Honda Hospital in San Francisco, California, is said to have been written by a ninety-year old woman in the geriatric ward of an English nursing home. It was discovered in her locker after she died, by staff members who thought she was incapable of writing.

What do you see, what do you see?
What are you thinking when you are looking at me?
A crabbed old woman, not very wise
Uncertain of habit, with faraway eyes
Who dribbles her food and makes no reply.
When you say in a loud voice, "I do wish you'd try."
I'll tell you who I am as I sit here so still,
I'm a small child of ten with a father and mother
Brothers and sisters who love one another;
A bride soon at twenty, my heart gives a leap
Remembering the vows that I promised to keep
At twenty-five now I have young of my own
Who need me to build a secure happy home.
At fifty once more babies play round my knee
Again we know children, my loved ones and me.
Dark days are upon me, my husband is dead
I look to the future and I shudder with dread
My young are all busy rearing young of their own
And I think of the years and the love I have known.
I'm an old woman now and Nature is cruel
'Tis her jest to make old age look like a fool.
The body crumbles, grace and vigour depart
There is now a stone where I once had a heart.
But inside this old carcass a young girl still dwells
And now and again my battered heart swells
I remember the joys; I remember the pain
And I'm loving and living all over again.
And I think of the years all too few... gone too fast
And accept the stark fact that nothing will last
So open your eyes, open and see,
Not a crabbed old woman; look closer... see me."

If your attention remains only on a person's physical condition, personality or mental state as you see or touch him or her, you will miss a unique opportunity to meet that person as an individual.

WILLINGNESS TO FACE DEATH

Gay Luce, a prominent teacher in the field of death and dying, once said that we put much more time and energy into getting ready for a trip to Hawaii than we do in preparing for our own death. This is particularly true in our Western culture where the fact of death is often hidden and denied as long as possible. This denial and lack of awareness seem odd since life itself is a terminal illness, so to speak, and death is a journey that every single one of us will take.

If we wish to support others in the dying process then I believe it is crucial to develop and practice something I would call death awareness or death preparation. We need to confront, to some degree, our own fears about death and dying. We need to have accepted the fact of our own mortality, to consciously experience the fact of death, to accept that death is a natural part of the life cycle and that we and everyone we love will one day die.

In my view, it is essential for those working in any capacity with the seriously or the "terminally" ill to identify personal areas of concern in relation to death and dying, to have some awareness of and to have processed to some extent, one's own fears about death. All training programs for hospice volunteers include such death awareness exercises and there are many other avenues available for looking at such issues.

Such processes should include opening your mind and heart to let your thoughts about death and dying surface, contemplating those fears until you have at least some understanding of where they come from or what they are based on, and communicating those fears to others. Such communications could be verbal and could also be expressed through written or artistic exercises. In my training workshops, one process I use to help participants access thoughts and feelings that may not yet have come into conscious awareness is a dyad technique in which participants give instructions to their partners such as:

Tell me a concern you have about aging.

Tell me a fear you have about death or dying.

Tell me what life is.

Tell me what death is.

You can do a form of this technique with a trusted friend or colleague. Decide on a topic and on a specific instruction to be given such as "Tell me a fear you have about aging," or "Tell me what death means to you." (See Appendix II for detailed instructions on how to do this exercise).

A formalized exercise such as the Dyad Communication Exercise can be a powerful and effective tool in accessing and processing your thoughts and feelings. The process works to the extent that you are able to honestly and completely express what occurs for you in regard to the particular issue you are working on and to the extent that you

One nurse took it upon herself to recommend my service to a daughter whose dad was in the facility. He was my first client and he became my walking advertisement. We became very close. He shared his regrets of life and vented his problems with staff with me. Then he would get a massage and calm right down... His sudden death hit me very hard and I had to deal with it which is one drawback of this type of work. I have come to realize that it's the quality of their time left that really makes the difference. It far outweighs the pain felt when they pass away.

ROSE GILMOUR, MASSAGE THERAPIST

I felt very sad leaving M's house after our touch session that day. I was fairly certain I would not see her again. It seemed so unfair for a woman her age—ten years younger than me—to be dying, and leaving behind a twelve-year-old daughter just at the time when she needed a mother so much! I took a wrong turn, or maybe several, and got completely lost coming back from my visit. Then I almost hit a huge truck. I had to stop the car and let myself cry before I could concentrate on getting home. When I finally got on the freeway, I rolled up all the car windows, turned on the radio and screamed my way to the exit.

AUTHOR

are able to open to and receive whatever another person communicates to you. An exercise such as this also gives you a chance to practice active listening skills. Much of our conversation in life is more casual. We are often interrupted or distracted and our thoughts are not always completed or fully understood by others. Listening without interrupting or commenting or offering advice (trying to "fix" something for the other person) provides a safe space for another to communicate what is true for him or her without fear of being judged or evaluated in any way. You can use this type of dyad format to work on almost any life issue where you feel "stuck", to improve your communication skills, and to deepen your contact with others.

Once you have begun your own self-inspection process in regard to illness, aging, death and dying, it will simply continue and deepen through your experience in service. You may well encounter new fears as you continue to work with people in later life stages (when you see someone with a particular deformity or suffering intense physical pain, for example). If you have developed some facility for facing and accepting your fears as they arise, then you will be able to keep your attention on the individual you are working with when your own anxiety and fears are awakened during a session. You can notice and acknowledge, rather than repress, deny or ignore your reactions, and go on with your session anyway. After the session you can look more closely at what occurred for you and work through what came up.

This process will begin to unfold more easily and more quickly until you hit a barrier, some new and previously denied personal experience with death (your own parent dying suddenly, a friend's child drowning or a life-threatening illness of your own, for example). Once you have confronted that particular barrier and moved through it, then you will simply continue on in your process at a deeper level.

As a touch practitioner working with those in later life stages, a volunteer caregiver or a family caregiver, you will be relating to people who are nearing the end of their lives. It will be helpful, therefore, for you to have some knowledge of the signs and symptoms of approaching death as outlined in the section *The Power of Touch in Caring for Our Dying*. You may be with another as he or she approaches this unique transition. You may actually be the only one present as that person breathes his or her last breath. The more acceptance and understanding you have of the death experience, the more support you can offer. You will be able to remain calm and alert, and keep your attention on the individual as you witness such a moment.

Stephen Levine said, in a workshop I once attended, that being with another human being at the moment of his or her death is a rare and wonderful opportunity, an experience to be welcomed because there is so much to learn from sharing in and witnessing such a significant event. I have found his statement to be profoundly true. I heard another teacher talk recently about feeling excited and even elated whenever he knows he is going to spend time with someone who is dying, because he knows he is going to be in the presence of Truth.

Touch Techniques

AGE-APPROPRIATE MASSAGE

People who are aging, ill and/or approaching death have varying degrees of tolerance for and responsiveness to touch. It is necessary to proceed with sensitivity and caution when administering therapeutic massage to such individuals. It is much better to begin with a focused but gentle touch and then gradually increase pressure, if it is requested or well tolerated, than to cause discomfort by starting with too much pressure.

Light pressure massage may be administered with the fingertips of both hands simultaneously almost anywhere on the body. The most common way to administer stronger pressure massage is probably with the thumbs. The entire upper back can be worked in this way, with the thumbs moving down the back simultaneously or in an alternating pattern, being careful never to press directly on the spine or on the scapula (shoulder blades).

Most often, pressure massage is combined with small circular thumb movements in a pattern covering an area such as the shoulders or back, but can also be used on the arch of the foot or palm of the hand. This technique may be used while working over clothing or directly on the skin.

Even quite elderly and fragile-looking people can often take medium to firm pressure on certain areas of the body such as the large trapezius muscles (which cross the tops of the shoulders) and the rhomboids (between the scapula and the spine).

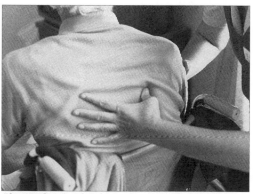

Photographer: Brock Palmer

I've started giving more lotion to my residents. I've got some residents who are comatose or really resistant to care. You touch them and they really resist you, don't want you. Since the workshop I've noticed when I've come to them and sat beside them and just kind of talked to them a little bit even though they couldn't talk back and just kind of touching their hand and they've started to reach out to me... one of my residents has started stretching her hand completely out and is raising it up so that I can get under it even better.

TERESA YATES, RESTORATIVE AIDE

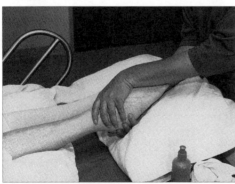

Photographer: Bonnie Burt

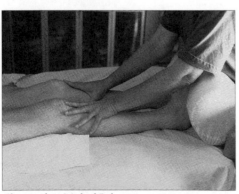

Photographer: Michael Pedersen

You can work on the rhomboid muscles with the thumbs by standing behind the back of a seated person. You can work on this same area with your fingertips by reaching underneath the shoulder and upper back while a person is lying face up in bed. Pressure massage may also be used with lotion, in which case the thumbs or fingertips, along with the whole hand on larger areas, would simply glide from one spot to the next without lifting off and the pressure would be continuous. Pressure may be applied with the thumbs moving down the back, either simultaneously or in an alternating pattern, on either side of the spine, with or without the use of lotion.

Squeezing, with light or medium pressure, can be done over clothing or even coverings like sheets or light blankets. It can also be done directly on the skin. Squeezing is usually accomplished with both hands simultaneously on extremities such as the legs or arms. This technique can best be described as opening and closing the hands around the body part being touched.

Moisturizing or "lotioning" is normally combined with stroking the body in some way and is done for one of two reasons. You may apply lotion for the purpose of adding moisture to the skin to relieve or prevent dryness. You might also apply lotion or oil as a skin lubricant, primarily for ease in massaging since it reduces friction. Suitable types of lubricants are discussed in the chapter entitled Touch Session Tools and Aids.

If the lotion you have has been exposed to cold and you have no way of warming it, then squeeze a small amount into the palm of your hand and rub them together vigorously a few times before bringing your hands into contact with the person's body. Avoid pouring or squeezing lotion or other lubricant directly onto anyone's body. A smooth cool lotion may, on occasion, feel refreshing to a fevered body. However, cold lotion, as well as cold hands, can be startling and uncomfortable.

Use lotion (or a combination of lotion and a little oil to thin the lotion if you think necessary) primarily for long massage strokes on the arms, legs or back. Keep the bottle close by (in an apron or massage belt or sitting on a nearby table) so that you can reach the container easily.

Some types of skin absorb moisture quite rapidly but other types do not need a lot of extra lubrication. Aging skin tends to absorb less quickly and other factors such as medications being taken can affect absorption as well. It is better to start with a little and add as needed rather than to have way too much lotion on the skin. Use just enough lotion so that your hands can glide easily and smoothly up and down the area you are stroking.

You can use lotion to moisturize drying or itching skin on the hands or feet or even parts of the face. Moisturize another's hands or feet with lotion the same way you would your own, covering the entire area well, using the palms and fingers of both your hands. Make sure you pay attention to the areas between fingers and toes. You can make a natural transition from moisturizing to massaging if the person is open to continued touching.

As you moisturize a foot, for instance, you can begin to gently squeeze with both hands around the middle part of the foot or with one hand around the heel. You might apply a little pressure with short up and down or circular strokes with your fingertips or with your thumbs on the arch of the foot. You might then move on up the leg to the knees, primarily applying lotion on the upstroke and letting your hands wrap around the leg so that they slide down the back side of the leg, applying a bit of pressure to the calf muscles with your fingertips as you slide down.

When you reach the ankle, you can repeat this leg stroke, using more lotion as you need it, or you can continue down over the foot with one hand on top and one on the bottom. You can apply this technique on one leg and foot at a time or on both legs at the same time.

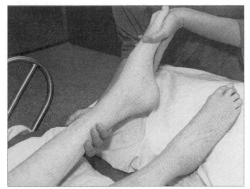
Photographer: Bonnie Burt

Similarly, as you moisturize a hand, you can move up onto the forearm with short strokes and, if the person seems receptive, go ahead and gradually moisturize and massage the rest of the arm. If you are sitting facing someone in a wheelchair (as described in the next chapter) with your chair positioned to the right side of the person's left arm, slip your left hand under the person's left hand and use your right hand to apply the lotion all the way up and down the left arm. To use the same technique on the person's right arm, you would position your chair to the left of the person's right side. This time, you would hold the person's right hand with your right hand, and with your left hand apply the lotion to his or her right arm. In both cases, let your hand mold itself to the shape of the person's arm and slide smoothly all the way up the arm and onto the top of the shoulder, circling around the shoulder and gliding down the back of the arm to the hand.

Another way of doing this moisturizing and massage stroke on the arm, especially if you are accessing the arm by standing beside a hospital bed, is to alternate your hands while working on the same arm. In other words, first support the person's hand and wrist with your right hand and let your left hand glide up the inside of the arm and back down, then support the person's right hand and wrist with your right hand and let your left hand do the moisturizing and stroking up and down the arm.

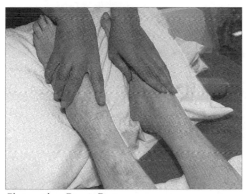
Photographer: Bonnie Burt

A stroke survivor I used to visit twice a month had, among other problems, only partial use of her right arm. In the beginning she wanted me to spend our whole session together just massaging her "bad" arm, although I always offered to do a little work on her other extremities. I eventually discovered that this lady was holding on to a belief that massage therapy was going to bring back the feeling in her arm. She frequently complained that I didn't come often enough and never spent enough time with her, thinking, I came to realize, that the more time I spent massaging her arm, the quicker her body would be back to "normal."

One day I offered to spend a little extra time with this resident and persuaded her to let me massage her other arm and her legs. I acknowledged the frustration she must be feeling about the loss of control over her physical body. I let her know that massage alone could not "heal" her paralysis. I told her some of the benefits I thought our sessions could provide, with her

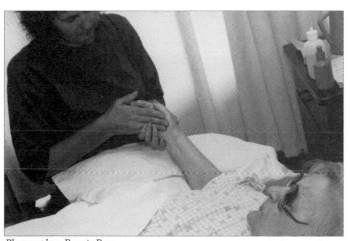
Photographer: Bonnie Burt

The first patient I was given as a new hospice volunteer was a woman whose body was riddled with cancer. I had been told that she would most likely be alive only a few more days. Her skin was pale but translucent and her eyes were large and beautiful in her thin face. She was weak and did not talk much, though she indicated that she enjoyed the gentle foot massage I gave her. I also moisturized her arms and hands with lotion. When I went back a couple of days later and asked if she'd like a foot massage, she said in a barely audible voice, "Let's just skip that today shall we?" I sat in a chair beside her bed while her husband went out to pick up a few groceries. I took one of her hands between both of mine and the two of us stayed together in this sacred silence for nearly twenty minutes. I kept my attention on her when her eyes were closed, and when they flickered open I simply met her gaze and continued holding her hand, conscious of our physical contact and aware of a deeper connection which was taking place.

AUTHOR

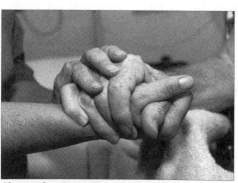

Photographer: Bonnie Burt

participation. I noticed that she seemed more relaxed and more willing to let me move on to visit other residents after I had touched both sides of her body, acknowledged the reality of her situation, and been honest with her about what our time together might and might not accomplish.

ATTENTIVE TOUCH

There will be times when the most compassionate thing you can do for another, in contacting that person on a physical level, is what might be called conscious, mindful or attentive touch. A person's body may simply be too sensitive or too traumatized to take any more pressure or movement than the gentlest of touches. Sometimes a person who is near death is becoming de-identified with the body and it is inappropriate to do anything other than hold a hand or make some other kind of gentle but conscious physical contact. This might be a soft touch with a fingertip or two at the top of the head or the bottom of the feet. It might be your hand on top of the bed covers gently molded around a wrist or ankle. The point is to be conscious of the physical connection as you make it. As you consciously and mindfully make the physical contact, you focus your awareness not just on the person's physical body, but on the individual whose body you are touching. Keep in mind that you are contacting that individual through the physical act of touch.

Taking a person's hand between both of yours as you hold that individual in your consciousness is an appropriate, reassuring and soothing form of touch. It is a one good way to begin a visit or a touch session. You can sense a great deal about a person's physical condition by holding his or her hand. You will be able to tell something about the person's strength and energy by the way in which that person responds to your touch. The temperature of the skin can give you an indication of how well the blood is circulating and about how active the person may be. You can pick up information about the person with this initial touch that will help you in deciding how to proceed in the touch session.

Actively holding one or both hands of the person you have been working with is also a good way to end a touch session. If you start the session with the hands, coming back to a similar simple touch after touching or massaging other parts of the body can bring a sense of completion and balance to your interaction with that individual in that particular session. If your relating has been verbal as well as physical, then sitting in silence for a few moments with your hands entwined can be calming and restful to both of you, although this cannot be forced. The person you are with may not necessarily feel comfortable in silence or may never stop talking.

There are also times when holding someone's hand between both of yours for an extended period of time may comprise the whole session. The person will derive benefit from your active physical connection as well as from your attention and your presence. The tender, loving touch of the human hand can be a powerful nonverbal communication. There are times when that touch alone is much more effective than any words we might say.

Even those who find a great deal of pleasure in being massaged and stroked may be unable to enjoy the same kind of physical contact they once did as their illness progresses and changes occur in their physical and mental state. You will need to adjust your touch accordingly and remain physically present, doing whatever seems to be comforting and supportive. You can try one hand resting gently on top of a person's head and the other hand over the heart.

Another comforting touch is holding one of the person's hands in one of yours while your other hand rests gently on his or her belly or chest.

You can effectively use attentive touch on other parts of the body as well. For example, you might stand behind a person sitting in a wheelchair and gently place both of your hands on the tops of her or his shoulders letting your fingers rest naturally over the front of the shoulders. In this case, you are not pressing down on the shoulders in any way. You are simply resting your hands on the body while keeping your attention on the person whose body you are contacting.

As you use this or other touch techniques, be aware of the energy moving through your body and out through your hands. Stay present with the individual whose body you are touching and stay awake to the energetic contact your touch creates. You can remain in this kind of contact for as long as you wish. When it seems appropriate, break the contact by allowing your hands to rise slowly up and away from the person's body. Allow a few moments for the effect of this contact to be absorbed before continuing with the same or another technique. You might also use this touch to the tops of the shoulders as the initial contact for a neck, shoulder and upper back massage.

The pressure you use with attentive touch can range from the very lightest contact to a fairly firm holding or enclosing. The amount of pressure you apply depends on the condition of the person's body, what you intuitively feel is appropriate, the positive and negative indicators that you observe, and the feedback you are receiving. If you are unsure of how much pressure to use and the person is able to respond either verbally or in some other manner, you can ask a direct question, "Am I pressing too hard?" or "Would you like me to press harder?" Avoid using "new age" or massage school phrasing such as "How's the pressure?" which may confuse the person unfamiliar with such jargon.

Lifting and Shifting

If you have ever been "felled" by a flu virus, recovered from a major physical trauma or surgical procedure or undergone treatments such as chemotherapy, you may recall or know firsthand what it feels like to be bedridden with an aching and weakened body. Sometimes it seems as if even moving to a different position on the bed would take more energy than you have available. Imagine being in such a situation for weeks or months! Skilled touch can provide welcome relief to muscles that ache from disuse or disease.

Sometimes actual touch or massage techniques can feel like too much stimulation in such a situation. Something as seemingly simple as consciously and gently lifting a leg or an arm and shifting it to a new

Repeatedly, I am awed that the most wondrous of all the massage strokes is that of simply 'resting'— resting my hands, resting my intentions, resting my heart as one would rest in contemplative prayer

MARY ANN FINCH, C.M.T.

A cancer patient whom I had been seeing for some weeks gradually lost feeling in most of her body. I continued to moisturize her skin and to do deeper massage on one arm and hand where she still had sensation. One day, at a loss as to what I could do that might be helpful to her, I stopped moving my hands and simply let them come to rest on her arm. As I sat beside her, remaining in physical contact and experiencing our connection, she surprised me by asking "What are you doing when you move around and then stop like that?" Since I had not been trying to "do" anything, I replied that I was simply remaining "in touch" with her. She responded, "Well, it's very calming."

AUTHOR

I recall placing my hands on top of the shoulders of a ninety-seven year old lady as she sat in her wheelchair in the hallway of the care facility where she resided. After talking with her for a few minutes, I had gone around behind her wheelchair. As I brought my hands gently into contact with her body, I felt her shoulders drop appreciably, and her whole body relax as a result of this simple touch. My relationship with this sweet, gracious and mentally alert lady continued until she died peacefully one day as she neared 100 years of age.

AUTHOR

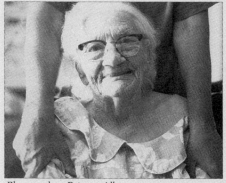

Photographer: Brianna Allen

position may be experienced by the person inhabiting that weakened body as merciful attention and relief.

When lifting legs or arms, be sure that you give adequate attention and support to the movement so that the person feels secure. In the case of a leg, put one hand under the heel or around the middle part of the foot and the other hand around the calf. Lift the leg a few inches, perhaps suspending it in air for a just a moment before gently lowering it back down onto the bed just an inch or two to the right or left of the previous spot where it lay.

Elevating the leg slightly by placing a small pillow or rolled-up towel under an ankle may help provide a needed shift in position (in addition to helping prevent pressure sores) for someone who is bedridden and too weak, or perhaps not cognizant enough to move a foot or leg by him or herself. Placing a bed pillow under the knees for awhile can often relieve strain on lower back muscles and help improve circulation.

Gently bending a straightened arm and placing a person's hand over his own heart or belly area can provide a positional shift and may also feel comforting. Raising someone's head slightly and placing a small pillow (or rolled-up towel) under the neck provides the weakened person with a moment of attentive touch and moves the neck muscles so that they don't become "frozen." Even raising the head enough to take out a bed pillow and letting the head lay back down on the bed while you shake out or fluff the pillow and then replace it under the head can provide a moment of relief.

You can lift the shoulder of a patient on his or her back off the bed as far as is comfortable for the patient and then let it rest again in its natural position. This movement can be repeated gently and slowly several times on each shoulder. While lifting the shoulder, you can reach under the upper back in order to do some circular stroking or fingertip pressure. If you are working directly on the skin, you can achieve a nice stroke on the back by moisturizing one hand with a bit of lotion, placing it under the upper back as you lift a shoulder, leaving it there after the shoulder is let down and then slowly pulling the hand out. Before touching any part of a person's body that you cannot see, you should ask or make sure that there is no wound, contagious rash or other skin condition that should not be touched.

Any body extremity that can tolerate gentle movement may be lifted off its resting place for a few moments in repeated sequences, giving the skin a rest, increasing body awareness and stimulating circulation. Gently stretching or pulling on an arm or leg can also feel good and this technique is easily combined with lifting and shifting.

MOTION AND MOVEMENT

Focusing attention on specific parts of the body increases body awareness in general. When people are too weak to move their own bodies, moving their limbs for them provides a form of mild exercise, which can improve circulation and stimulate the brain. In a manner of speaking, the movement is like "oiling the joints" in the body so that they don't get rusty. Unless you are a physical or occupation therapist, or working under the guidance of such a person, you should avoid doing any "range of motion" work. You can however, assess a person's limitations and encourage movement by asking such questions as "How high can you raise this arm?" or "Can you move this hand?" Always let people initiate movement on their own if they are able to do so. This will give them a sense of control, progress and accomplishment while increasing their body awareness.

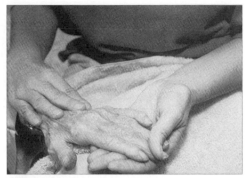

Photographer: Bonnie Burt

Small, gentle movement may be used in a massage or touch session to explore motion in the joints. Fingers, wrists, ankles, arms and legs, or any other part of the body connected by joints may be gently moved in small circles, up and down or from side to side. Just being reminded that a part of the body still works can bring a smile to the face of someone who has been inactive or immobile for a while or who has "forgotten" to move. Be sure that you leave any specific physical therapy techniques to those who have been trained to perform such tasks.

One of my first clients was a nursing home resident in her late nineties who could no longer walk and spent most of her waking hours in a wheelchair. She was a sweet, white-haired elderwoman with a beautiful and ready smile. She loved having her hands massaged. One day, I noticed her watching me intently as I held one of her hands in both of mine and, using lotion and a gentle squeezing massage technique, worked slowly over her whole hand, gently massaging each finger from the base to the tip. As I went on to her other hand, she raised her arm off her lap and brought the palm of her right hand up close to her eyes. She began wiggling her fingers in seeming wonder and surprise, smiling and chuckling to herself. Then I heard her say, "I didn't know I could do that!"

Whatever techniques you are using, always touch both sides of the body so that you leave the person with a sense of balance and completeness in terms of your attention and of the physical stimulation and body awareness which your touch initiates. This principle applies even if the person has no feeling in one side of the body. If a leg or arm is missing, you can touch or massage whatever part is still there if the person is comfortable with your doing so.

PSYCHIC TOUCH

There may come a time when even the most sensitive massage is too much or when even the gentlest touch becomes almost intolerable to someone with whom you have been working. If even very light physical contact is uncomfortable for the person, you can still apply what I might call "psychic touch" with your loved one, patient or client by holding him or her in your consciousness, maintaining contact through your physical presence and your attention. In other words, you stay mentally connected to the individual and in close physical proximity, with all your senses attentive to both the body and the being you are with. That person will experience your presence on some level. Your conscious attention offers comfort and support so that she or he feels less isolated and alone.

You can also direct your attention to a specific area of a person's body where he or she is experiencing pain even if it is not possible to

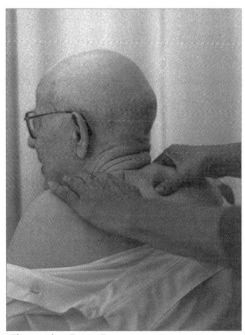

Photographer: Bonnie Burt

actually touch that area, which may be bandaged or in a cast, for example. Holding your hands directly above an area of the body that is swollen, discolored, inflamed, bruised or contracted can sometimes be enough to bring some degree of relief to the person in pain. You could hold your hands just above the area and send your energy there. If a person is alert, I sometimes say "Well, let's both just send our love to that spot." In this way two people have their attention on the place that hurts and sometimes that action and that energy can provide relief. The person then relaxes just a little, perhaps breathes a bit easier and the discomfort is reduced at least momentarily.

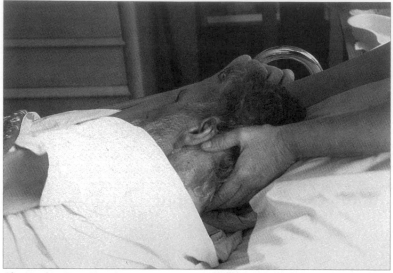

Photographer: Barry Barankin

While your attention is directed toward the area of the body in pain, you can validate the fact of the person's injury or physical trauma by a simple verbal acknowledgment such as "I'm sorry." Those two words, along with your focused energy and attention, have enormous power. The individual feels seen, feels acknowledged, and experiences a moment of compassion and caring from another individual. The person recognizes that he or she does not have to bear the pain all alone, that another individual is willing to "receive" it. Such an understanding may precipitate a shift in the person's perceptions about the discomfort and this change in thinking may alter the way he or she experiences the pain.

I had a classmate once who was given an assignment, along with the rest of us, of spending two hours a week with someone who was near death. She went to her local nursing home and asked if there was anyone there whom she might visit in order to fulfill this class requirement. The activity director denied that anyone in that facility was near death, seeming to take the assumption that there might be someone there fitting such a description as a personal affront. When my classmate persisted, she finally said that there was a nonresponsive woman at the end of the hall who apparently never had any visitors and that she could sit with her if she wished. My classmate encountered this woman, isolated and alone in the last room by the exit door in a long hallway. The woman was curled up in a fetal position on her bed, clothing and hair in disarray. My classmate felt ill equipped to help this rather pitiful-looking person. However, she had agreed to spend the time there. She decided that she would not try to talk to or touch this woman. What she did was simply sit down on a chair near the bed and put her attention on the woman. She did this twice a week for about an hour each visit. After a few sittings, the woman in the bed turned her body toward my friend and came slightly out of her fetal position. After a few more visits, she turned her head, and eventually she opened her eyes to look at this person who was doing nothing other than keeping her attention on her. By this time, my classmate felt herself to be in a relationship with the woman and so she experienced this response as quite miraculous.

Accessing Bodies in Wheelchairs and Beds

M any elderly people in care facilities spend a good deal of time sitting in wheelchairs. This section outlines ways to access the bodies of such people for the purpose of offering a touch session which might include lotioning or massaging the hands and arms as well as the shoulders and upper back. There are a number of different models of wheelchairs. I have yet to see one that looks as though it would be comfortable to sit in for long periods of time. Some have higher or lower backs, wider or narrower arm rests and so on. Some wheelchairs are designed so that the sides can be easily removed, which makes accessing the arms much easier.

The important thing is for both you and the person you are touching to be comfortable. You may need to make adjustments to these suggestions or create ways that work for you in any given situation.

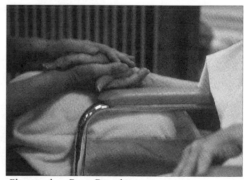

Photographer: Barry Barankin

1. **Sitting in straight-back chair or stool placed adjacent to wheelchair**

   a. Mirror image placement: facing the person in the wheelchair on either side of chair, to access hands, arms and shoulders. Use a pillow to equalize space between your laps or slip your arm underneath the arm of the person in the wheelchair, cradling his or her elbow in the palm of your hand. Do not use a pillow on the arm of the wheelchair as this will push the person's shoulder up into a contracted position.

   b. Perpendicular placement of your chair to the wheelchair to reach upper arms, opposite shoulder and upper back.

2. **Standing**

   a. Side lunge position on either side of wheelchair: leaning your body against the wheel or straddling the wheel to access opposite side of the back or to go down to the lower back.

   Note: If you have the person lean forward in order to access the lower back, have him or her hold onto a pillow, if possible, and then use one arm across that person's chest to give him or her a feeling of safety and comfort. The person does not need to lean far forward—only a couple of inches

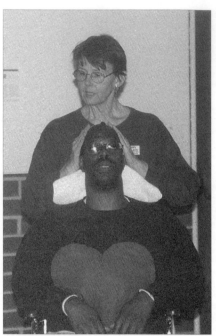

Photographer: Shawnee Isaac-Smith

   b. Standing behind chair (knees slightly bent) to access the head and shoulders or to move down both arms at the same time.

   Note: If using rolled-up towel or neck roll pillow behind the person's head (as described on pages 111–112), make sure the head is only slightly angled back (as illustrated in the photograph).

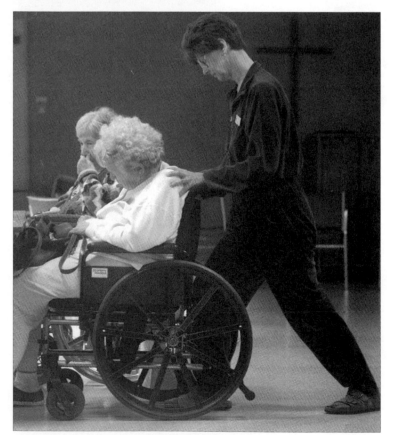

Photographer: Karl Mondon

3. Kneeling

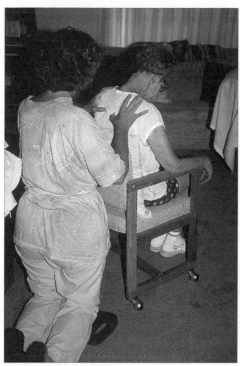

Photograph: Barry Barankin

a. One knee on pad at either side of wheelchair, or behind the chair (as illustrated in the photograph).

b. Both knees on pad, sitting on legs in front of chair to access feet and legs.

Note: If you have no kneepad you could use a towel or pillow. Make sure you have something to cushion and protect your knees!

If the person with whom you are doing a touch session is in a hospital or home bed, you can position your chair at the side of the bed or possibly sit or stand at the end of the bed to access the feet and legs. Occasionally a bed in the home will be on rollers and can be easily moved. If so, you can stand at the other end of the bed in order to reach the head, face, neck and shoulders. In most facilities, however, moving the bed is not an option, so you must simply find a way to position your body that is comfortable for both you and the person you are touching.

Remember that you can raise or lower hospital beds. This gives you more options and allows you to work more comfortably. There are a number of different mechanisms for accomplishing this and I've had to ask someone more than once over the years to show me how to lower a bed rail. If a height adjustment is not possible or if you sense that the sound and movement would be too jarring to the person in the bed, then you must adjust your own height. You can try placing blankets or pillows on your chair, possibly sitting on the bed with the person, getting down on your knees on a kneepad, or whatever works and does not make your or the person you are touching uncomfortable!

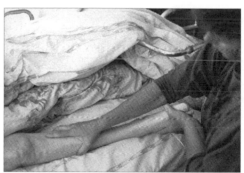

Photographer: Barry Barankin

Touch Session
Aids and Tools

The most important gift you have to give another is your self. You need bring nothing else to a touch session. There are, however, some practical items which can be helpful when used as aids in conjunction with your presence, your inner resources and touch techniques. If you are caring for someone at home, or if you are a healthcare professional who has chosen to offer a massage or touch session as a special and separate activity, you might want to gather a few of these items together and keep them in one place so that they are handy when you need them. If you are a massage practitioner providing massage or skilled touch as an outreach service, you will want to purchase some kind of tote bag to hold the items you may need and carry it with you to your sessions.

In some situations and for certain massage techniques, lubrication will be needed. When I first began working with those in later life stages, I tried the same kind of massage oil I was used to using with clients who came to my home studio and stretched out on my massage table. With those clients, I usually heated the oil before beginning a massage session. This practice did not transfer well to the nursing home setting. After a short time, I quit using oil with the frail elderly and the seriously ill for several other reasons:

- Older people respond much more positively to lotion. To most of them, oil is something you cook with, not something you put on your skin.
- Oil is more difficult to work with because you need two hands to use it.
- The skin of aged and ill people often does not absorb the oil well.

The kind lotion you choose to use is simply a matter of preference for you and for the people you are working with. You can experiment with different products until you find a few you particularly like. The lotion needs to be thin enough to glide well and feel smooth and soothing to the skin.

Hospitals sometimes supply lotions to patients but I have found that those products tend to be "sticky" and not the most suitable for use in moisturizing or massaging. I usually bring a couple of different containers of lotion to a touch session. On more than one occasion, however, I have had an older woman tell me to "save" my lotion and use the one that is there because it is "free." If the person prefers that I use the lotion provided, or one which she or he has on hand, then I do so.

It is good to have at least one scented and one unscented lotion on hand. If you are administering touch sessions to someone on a regular basis, he or she may develop a preference for a particular lotion and ask for it. This happened to me with a hospice patient who became so attached to a specific product that I, along with her family members, began to "stock up" on it so that it would be available at all times. It was a good thing we did so because at some point the company changed the formula and the lotion in its original form was suddenly no longer available.

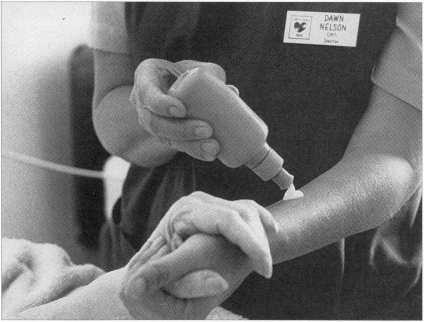

Photographer: Bonnie Burt

It is best to have a pump or squeeze-type container for your lotion so that you do not have to let go of someone's hand or interrupt your touch in order to get more lotion. You can squeeze some lotion onto your own forearm as illustrated above and access it as needed to moisturize the hand and are you are holding

You can set a pump-type container on a nearby table or shelf, or on the floor by your chair so that you can simply reach out or down with your free hand to replenish your supply of lotion.

Unless I am combining aromatherapy with a touch session, I've found it is usually best to start with a lotion that has only a very mild fragrance or none at all, unless someone makes a specific request. Some older people have a heightened sense of smell and find strong scents overpowering or unpleasant. Those who are ill may be particularly sensitive to odors or may feel temporary aversions to certain fragrances that did not bother them in the past. This may be especially true of people who are undergoing radiation or chemotherapy treatments. If I

sense that someone might prefer a scented lotion, I let that person smell it before I apply it and gauge the response. This interaction helps build rapport and gives the person some control in the situation.

If you discover particularly dry skin on the hands or feet, you may want to use a heavier body lotion or a cream such as Eucerine, which can be purchased in almost any drug or grocery store. If someone has arthritis, you can apply an analgesic cream or gel formulated to relieve that particular discomfort. Always let an alert person know what you are using – read the label out loud or let the person read it— and make sure it is okay with him or her. The fact that you have noticed

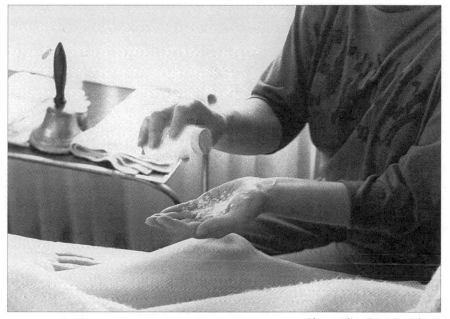

Photographer: Barry Barankin

the condition and offered something special tends to make the person feel acknowledged and cared for, and helps build trust.

Powder applied to the skin can feel soothing and comforting to some people. There are those who prefer it to the feel of lotion on their skin. Dry powder is easily applied and can contribute to a feeling of being nurtured and taken care of. It is sometimes helpful to apply powder to areas of the body that tend to collect moisture or do not get exposure to air, such as underneath large breasts or between the toes. There may be times when you will want to use powder for specific problems, as an alternative to a moisturizer, or just for a change.

Cornstarch-based powders are preferable to talc if there is any chance of an ill person breathing talc into the lungs. A sample or travel-size container of powder will last for some time.

A few small hand towels can prove quite useful during a touch session. You can roll up a small towel and put it under an ankle or wrist to elevate a foot or arm for easier access, or to allow for better circulation. You can spread a hand towel over a small pillow on top of your lap before placing someone's arm on it. You might use the towel for wrapping around a foot to warm it or for removing any excess lotion that may not have absorbed into the skin. I have on occasion used a towel over a bedside rail for help in gripping and also to wipe up a spill or leakage.

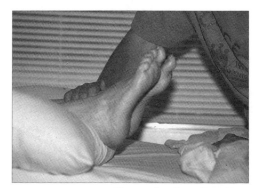

Photographer: Barry Barankin

A small tubular-shaped neck pillow can also be a helpful accessory. Some people like it as a change from the larger bed pillow or it can be used to give added support to a person's neck by putting it on top of the

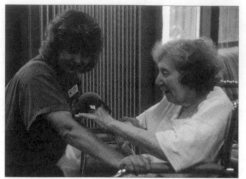

Photographer: Barry Barankin

bed pillow. If you are standing behind a chair or a wheelchair, you can put the pillow between the person's neck and your body and encourage him or her to relax against it (as shown in the photograph on page 106). If someone's head falls to one side or the other, the pillow can be used for support between the head and the shoulder. The neck pillow can also provide support under an ankle or knee while you are working. It is more easily negotiated than a large bed pillow, which may or may not be available. You can make neck pillows yourself or find them in various catalogs and stores. (I find I tend to give them away on a fairly regular basis!)

You might want to keep on hand a small container (not a roll-up tube) of some kind of salve or balm for applying to parched and chapped lips. Eucerine can also be applied for this purpose. One caregiver I know, whose husband had chronic chapping on his lips said Eucerine was the best thing she ever found to help this problem. If the person you are working with needs assistance, use your fingertip to apply the salve and remember to wash your hands before and after such applications.

I have found it useful to wear an apron with pockets (such as those worn by waiters or beauticians) especially when I am going to be seeing different people consecutively. The apron protects your clothing and gives you an easy place to keep your lotion and other small items, so that these things are always with you and easily accessed as you need them. Such aprons are not costly and come in a variety of colors and materials. Beauty supply and restaurant supply houses are one source for these aprons, or you could make your own. There is also a product on the market called a massage holster—something similar to a carpenter's belt except that it has only one or two loops for carrying bottles of lotion. A pump-type bottle of lotion fitted into such a belt will free your hands and allow easy and quick access to the lubricant as you work, if you are standing up. It tends to be cumbersome if you are sitting or kneeling.

If you are working as a volunteer or as a professional caregiver or as a service provider in care facility settings, you will need to have an identification badge or label so that people will know who you are and what you do. Seeing your name in writing as well as hearing it helps people remember it. If you are part of a volunteer organization you will probably be issued a permanent name badge or a temporary sticker to write your name on each time you visit. Make sure that your name is printed in letters large enough to be easily read and that there is not too much information, which might be confusing. An identification badge may be especially helpful for individuals you work with who are hard of hearing or nonverbal.

None of these items is absolutely essential for a touch session. I have found frequent uses for most of them over the years, however, and I like to have them with me or nearby. They will all fit easily into a medium-sized canvas tote bag which you can keep in a closet for home use or near your front door or in your car, so that it is easily accessible for visits to facilities or elsewhere.

I have found that diaper bags work quite well for use as touch session totes. They usually have several pockets that are perfect for bottles of lotion and room for a couple of hand towels and a small pillow. They come in many different colors and materials and have convenient shoulder straps.

There are a few other things that I usually carry with me when I'm going to give a touch session. I take several soft animal finger puppets which I sometimes use to help build rapport with people who are less verbal or have dementia and for those who may be shy about accepting direct physical contact. They have proven useful as communication aids with some people. One lady used to speak to the puppet on my finger in a different voice than she normally used and say things to the puppet that she never said to me directly. The particular puppet I first showed her happened to be a beaver and it also stimulated her long-term memory, reminding her of the television show *Leave It to Beaver* and of a particular time in her life. I always have at least two of these little critters with me in case someone wants one on his or her hand so that we can have a two-way animal conversation! I have also used these furry friends for tactile and sensory stimulation, and every once in awhile I leave one with a resident who seems to really enjoy using it or who is reluctant for me to end a session.

Another item that I have found to be almost indispensable over the years is a kneeling pad. These lightweight knee savers, the kind used for gardening, can be purchased in most plant nurseries. Some are made of foam and can be machine washed; other pads have a heavier rubber or vinyl covering. They measure about 15" by 7" and come in a variety of colors. Mine fits easily into my tote bag where I can find it quickly and easily. Dropping the kneepad on the floor enables me to kneel beside a wheelchair or bed if an extra chair is not available, giving me better access to the person I'm going to be touching and often making it possible for me to be at approximately the same eye level with that person. It also cushions and protects my knees from the hard floor, making it much more comfortable to be in the kneeling position.

Complimentary Relaxation Techniques

AROMATHERAPY

One day, when visiting a woman in a nursing home whom I'd been seeing twice a month for a couple of years, I took in a gift someone had given me labeled "Peppermint Foot Lotion." This particular resident loved the smell and wanted me to use it on her shoulders and neck where the fragrance would linger and she could enjoy it for awhile. From that day on, as soon as I walked in the room, she would ask me if I brought the "special" lotion. I soon bought more to make sure I always had some and gave her another container to keep by her bedside.

One day, I let another lady in the same facility, whom I'd known for years, smell this lotion and she said immediately, "Oh that reminds me of something!" She kept inhaling the peppermint scent, in obvious enjoyment as I encouraged her (thinking to myself that she surely must be trying to retrieve some memory having to do with Christmas and candy canes) when she suddenly exclaimed "Summertime! It reminds me of summertime!" Apparently, for this lady, the scent had more to do with ice cream than Christmas.

I have never enrolled in a formal study of aromatherapy (the art and science of using essential oils from natural botanicals to promote health and well-being). However, after these two incidents, I began to

*Aromatherapy in the hospice setting
can be extremely helpful for care of
the skin, mood stabilization, pain
management and the connection
with the spiritual aspects of being.*

LARAINE KYLE, C.N.S.,
AROMATHERAPIST

*Aromatic herbs have been used since
antiquity to cleanse and heal both
body and mind.*

SHIRLEY PRICE, AROMATHERAPY FOR
COMMON AILMENTS

experiment with using various scents as a way of stimulating memory and as a tool for enhancing relaxation during touch sessions. Around this same time I read about a small study conducted by Meghan Carnarius, an R.N. and an aromatherapist working in a nursing home in Boulder, Colorado. Ms. Carnarius found aromatherapy to be helpful in caring for those with dementia in the following ways:

- calming those who were agitated
- stimulating those who were lethargic
- promoting better sleep for those with insomnia

Ms. Carnarius stated that her objective was "to improve the quality of patients' lives" and that "Smell can make patients feel connected to their senses and therefore connected to their humanity."[34] She also pointed out that adding pleasant aromas to the normally static nursing home environment can affect the overall mood.

I had recently taken over the running of a massage program, which a former student and colleague had begun at a local nusring home. The administrator at the facility had known Meghan Carnarius in Boulder and seen first-hand the beneficial effects of aromatherapy in the nursing home setting. She provided a budget for the supplies and I brought in another former student, Chris Bailey, who was knowledgeable in this area and eager to integrate aromatherapy into the touch sessions already being provided to a group of residents. Chris created the blends mentioned below. Staff members were encouraged to use this new resource as well.

SUGGESTIONS FOR AROMATHERAPY USAGE

Blends:

1. **Stress/Calming** (use for agitation, irritability, restlessness, and for comfort)

2. **Clarity/Memory** (use for confusion, disorientation)

3. **Purify/Detox** (use for disinfecting, strengthening and for illness)

4. **Energize/Revitalize** (use for fatigue, depression, boredom)

5. **Refresh/Uplift** (use for refreshment, encouragement, pleasure)

Application:

1. **Air Mist**

   Put a few drops of essential oil in a water-filled spray bottle.

   Use the spray bottle for the immediate vicinity, or spray directly on the skin (avoid face).

2. **Dermal**

   Add a drop of oil to lotion in your hand or several drops to a small bottle of lotion and apply after bathing, for hand massage activity or as a special treat.

3. **Inhalation**

    Using a small dropper bottle, apply 3–5 drops on cotton ball, pillow case or tissue tucked into a shirt or sweater pocket.

    Caution: Do not hand a scented tissue directly to a resident.

4. **Environmental scenting with ScentBall®**

    Use in resident's room, hallways or at nursing station

    Use as an intervention before behavior problems manifest, if possible. For a small to medium-size room, apply 6–10 drops to pad. Insert pad in ScentBall®. Plug into any electrical outlet for up to one hour. (If left much longer, there is no fire hazard but an unpleasant smell may develop). To replace pad, simply push the new one in and the old one will come out.

    Note: If using dropper bottles, replace caps immediately to avoid spills. If a pure essential oil is accidentally rubbed in eyes, use whole milk eye wash or wipe eyes with a mild vegetable oil.

During the winter holiday season, Chris made up a special aromatherapy blend that filled the hallways and was enjoyed by residents and family members alike. The director of the Alzheimer's unit in the facility made use of a kitchen in the unit to promote what he called "natural aromatherapy" by baking cookies, chocolate cake, popping popcorn and so on, which was very effective in drawing the attention of many of the residents, stimulating memory, and creating opportunities for reminiscing. Flowers and fruits can be used in a similar way.

I have since seen a number of articles and studies, particularly coming out of Canada and Great Britain, on the successful clinical use of aromatherapy in Alzheimer's programs, dementia centers, intensive care units, hospices and other healthcare environments. Benefits cited include assistance in reducing high anxiety levels in a woman with a long history of mental illness, quieting a noisy room full of patients, and reducing the need for both pain-relieving and sedating medications. The Integrated Care Programme for Patients Living with Cancer at the Royal London Homeopathic Hospital enhances the effect of conventional cancer treatments by using aromatherapy along with a wide "range of other complimentary therapies including homeopathy, reflex zone therapy... visualisation and acupuncture"[35]

Aromatherapy can be easily combined with touch, in several different ways, to induce as well as enhance relaxation. Interest in clinical aromatherapy is continuing to grow and expand within the holistic health field. For more information on aromatherapy and its usage contact the National Association for Holistic Aromatherapy, or consult one of the following books:

- *Aromatherapy for Common Ailments* by Shirley Price, Simon & Schuster, 1991
- *The Aromatherapy Book: Applications and Inhalations* by Jeanne Rose, North Atlantic Books, 1992

Music... contributes not only to the relaxation of the body, but also to the healing of the spirit.

CHARLES GOURGEY,
HOSPICE VOLUNTEER

...when I sat and listened to music I forgot all about the pain.

IDA GOLDMAN, AGE 90,
TESTIFYING AT A SENATE HEARING,
8 JANUARY 2001

F was a hospice patient who enjoyed her massage sessions tremendously. She was also being seen regularly by the music therapist and felt greatly helped by their time together as well. It was one of F's fondest dreams that the music therapist and I might one day come and see her at the same time. We arranged for this to happen and I felt we all three received great benefit from this hour of music and massage. It seemed as if we had become one cohesive unit as the music therapist played a haunting and mesmerizing flute sonata and I slowly stroked and moisturized the patient's arms and legs.

AUTHOR

MUSIC

Music seems to have a special power to affect consciousness and sound can have a profound effect on the nervous system. The ancient Greeks believed that music could be used to heal. They played zithers as an aid to digestion and other instruments to induce sleep and to treat mental disturbances. Many contemporary practitioners of holistic healthcare use music in working with their clients, as part of the therapeutic process. There are several good books on the market today which detail, both theoretically and experientially, the benefits and effects of music in a healing process.

I have seen music used in a variety of ways to great effect in Alzheimer's programs and in what is sometimes called "end of life care." Music is now used as a therapeutic tool in many cancer centers and hospice programs; and other options for utilizing music as an aid in healing are being explored and researched

Sound and music can be used quite effectively in tandem with skilled touch and massage to help facilitate communication and relaxation. Both music and massage can help bring temporary relief from pain and induce a relaxation response. Both can stimulate memory and relieve despondency. Both can decrease anxiety and restlessness and can aid in improving the quality of sleep. Both can help enhance quality of life and can help ease the transition into death.

A music therapist friend of mine who works with hospice patients has successfully used a variety of tools for pain reduction and relaxation. He talks about the efficacy of certain techniques as an alternative to costly medications:

> *I use music and vibrational touch to relieve pain. One patient of mine had severe arthritic pain. I placed large tuning forks on her joints. The forks massaged the tissue with a very high but mild frequency. At the same time, she listened to relaxing nature sounds in the same frequency as the tuning fork. Afterward, she was pain free and able to move around for three days without the help and limitations of drugs.*[36]

It is clear that certain kinds of music can enhance the relaxation experience, though the same music does not work with every person, and different music may be appropriate at different times even with the same person. If you sense that listening to a specific piece of music might be helpful to someone you are relating to through touch, do not hesitate to suggest playing it, either during or after your touch session with that person.

Although music need not be an integral part of a massage or touch session, it can greatly enhance the therapeutic process. It is not likely to be detrimental in any way, although sometimes silence during a session is preferable or more appropriate. If you have a loved one or client who is a musician or music lover, you may want to consider contacting a music therapist who specializes in working with the elderly or the seriously ill.

I have, on occasion, purposely brought a cassette tape recorder and tapes with me to a touch session, and played a particular piece of music in order to help facilitate the relaxation process in working with certain individuals or to facilitate increased rapport with that person. For example, I used to visit a gentleman who was blind. I discovered through our conversations that he loved jazz music; and I found that he became much more relaxed, less distracted and more open to touch therapy when I put on a Benny Goodman or a Jimmy Dorsey tape during our sessions.

Occasionally someone may find music that he or she had previously enjoyed unpleasant or irritating. Sometimes a person's hearing becomes acutely sensitive and that person finds almost any sound becomes annoying. Even talking may, at some stage, become jarring to the psyche. In such cases, it is best just to sit with a person, touching her or him in whatever natural way seems appropriate to the moment, and maintaining a silent connection through touch and eye contact, when possible.

For some weeks before my grandmother died, she frequently made a humming sound almost like a chant. Before this time she had often enjoyed hearing me sing to her or listening to a tape of me singing or reading. At this point, however, it seemed to me that she was making her own music, so to speak, and that to impose other sounds on her would be intrusive and disrupting. It was obvious that the sound she was making was comforting to her and it seemed to be happening spontaneously. I have occasionally walked into convalescent facilities and heard a virtual chorus of singing, chanting and "sounding" from residents.

A hospice patient I'd been working with for some weeks was growing increasingly weak and was preparing to die. He was an accomplished musician and a lover of music. On this particular day his caregiver had put on a tape recording of a pianist playing as beautifully as anyone I've ever heard. As I sat with this individual, administering very gentle touch therapy and breathing with him in those precious moments, the sweetness of the music seemed to fill the room and enfold us until it felt as if we both disappeared inside of the sound. It was an experience I will never forget. While listening to his favorite opera a few days later, this gifted, gentle man slipped quietly out of his body during the last act.

RESOURCES

For further information on music as a therapeutic modality and its applications in healthcare settings, contact:

> The National Association for Music Therapy, Inc.
> 8455 Colesville Road, Ste. 1000
> Silver Spring, MD 20910
> Phone: 301-589-3300   Fax: 301-589-5175
> info@musictherapy.org

For information on programs dedicated to providing music to ease the dying experience, contact:

> Chalice of Repose Project at St. Patrick's Hospital
> 312 East Pine Street
> Missoula, MT 59802
> Phone: 406-329-2810   Fax: 406-329 5614

When working with hospice patients, whether conscious or unconscious, I usually use soothing music on a cassette player or hum to a patient just to let them know I'm there and happy to be working with them. It's very relaxing to them to do the massage or apply lotion to the soothing beat of the music or in soothing slow motions.

SHERRY PUYLLEY, HOME HEALTH AIDE

A patient of mine, afflicted with AIDS was taking high doses of morphine daily. She chose to replace the morphine with vibrational relaxation. I taught her how to apply tuning forks to places on her skin which would affect nerve centers. She continued the practice daily, with my help once a week, for a year and a half. She is now pain free without painkillers or morphine, enjoys her life and has saved thousands of dollars in pharmaceutical costs.

STEPHAN BETZ, PhD, MT-BC

VISUALIZATION

Creative visualization, forming pictures or images in the mind's eye, works quite well as both an affirmation and a relaxation technique for some people. Guiding or directing someone in creating images in the mind is a technique which has been widely and successfully used as an aid in pain control and stress management, for fostering self-awareness, and as a psychological tool or process leading to deeper insight and clarity. The number of commercially produced cassette tapes now on the market which contain guided fantasies and visualization exercises attest to the popularity and accessibility of this modality. I know many people who use such tapes as a sleep-inducing aid, for support in pain and stress control and to help achieve deep states of peace and relaxation. The success of this type of technique is a powerful indicator of how thoughts influence both physical and emotional states.

The dimension of touch, along with the voice of a real and accessible person can escalate the benefits of a guided visualization technique. You may assist an individual through the use of guided visualization, for instance, in becoming aware of his or her breath and breathing patterns. You may be able to help someone move from shallow chest breathing to a deeper and more relaxing abdominal or belly breathing. You can direct a person's attention to specific parts of the body as you are touching or massaging that part by giving a verbal instruction to bring his or her attention to that place.

If I am with an ill or an aged person who is mentally alert enough to follow my directions, I sometimes ask that person if he or she is willing to try something a little different, something that is sometimes used to help people relax. It is important to keep in mind that someone eighty or older is not likely to be familiar with "new age" relaxation techniques and that such processes may seem strange, awkward, or even ridiculous!

If the person is "game," then I might try asking him or her to visualize "untying" a knotted muscle while I gently massage the tight spot. Or, I tell the person to imagine that his or her breath is a particular color and then direct the person to send the breath into the tense area. I might try asking someone to imagine his or her tension or tightness as a hard block of ice, and then guide that person in visualizing the ice dissolving or becoming liquid. Another image that sometimes works well is that of a rope with many knots which turns into a ribbon of smoke. You can make up any image that you sense might work for a particular individual. When you find the right image, the results can be almost magical. Be sure to point out to those you work with in this manner that they can use such techniques on their own, without you. Never abuse people by making them think that you are the one "doing" the relaxing or creating the change in state that they experience.

You could also use guided fantasy or visualization techniques as a stress-reducing or calming device by helping a person to create a tranquil and beautiful scene of some kind in the mind's eye, a peaceful space or place where that person feels comfortable, safe and happy. If you are able to ascertain through asking questions or through written records something about a person's life before incapacitation, you may be able to find something to use as a jumping off place in creating such a fantasy. If the person was an expert mountain climber, for instance, you could start with that image. If you know that someone enjoyed vacationing in Hawaii every year, you could begin a guided visualization by asking that person to imagine her or himself walking along a seashore, feeling the warm sun beaming down and the sand under foot. You could go on to guide that person in mentally creating an idyllic island scene. Be sure to have the person visualize him or herself in the scene. Encourage the person you are working with in this way to add to the scene anything he or she might desire to make the place or the situation perfect in every way—favorite foods, flowers, weather, other people or animals, etc.

Most people who enjoy this technique are eventually able to visualize their "special place" without a voice guiding them. They can then create their ideal scene any time they chose and experience themselves relaxing into the peaceful, contented state which the scene evokes. As an interim solution you might make a tape recording of your voice for those who do well with the process, if they have access to a tape recorder and are able to use it.

In the case of the alert aged, you can use a visualization technique as both a relaxation process and as a reminiscence tool or as an aid in creating oral histories. I have watched aged individuals take on youthful characteristics as they re-live important events in their lives by talking about them to someone who cares enough to listen. Their eyes start to sparkle, color comes to their skin and they become animated and cheerful as they are encouraged to expand on happy memories, talk about career accomplishments or share some special experience.

You might ask a person to close his or her eyes and concentrate on the inhalation and exhalation of the breath as you administer a foot massage. After the person begins to relax, ask him or her to remember a particularly happy or important event (or one when the person felt the strongest, most proud, etc.). You can guide and encourage someone in re-creating a scene and then help that person expand the scene to include sense memory by asking specific questions about the time of year, the weather, colors, sights, sounds and so on. In effect, you are working on improving a person's circulation on the physical level, while that person is improving his or her mental and emotional circulation, so to speak, through this type of visualization and sense memory process.

GUIDED MEDITATION AND EXPLORATION

Meditation is a means of directing thought or focusing attention, of bringing conscious awareness to each moment as it arises. The practice itself can be something as simple as keeping one's attention concentrated on one's own breath, focusing on the flame of a candle as it burns, or consciously repeating a meaningful word or words.

Guided meditations, which use spoken words as a focus for the mind, can be used in conjunction with administering touch therapy. Such a tool is especially helpful if you are working with someone who is

One lady I worked with in an assisted care facility was always very quiet as I moisturized and massaged her extremities. One day I asked her what kinds of things she used to like to do and her whole countenance changed as she immediately responded, "Dancing!" I asked her questions about what kind of dancing, who she went dancing with, what her favorite music was, etc. until she had painted a "moving" picture for me of her nights out on the town in San Francisco with her girlfriends. I had a fuller understanding of this elderly woman's life and she found pleasure in re-creating and sharing those memories with me.

AUTHOR

I was sitting by the bedside of R whom I'd become quite fond of in the relatively short time we had spent together. The illness he had fought for two years had finally wasted his body and he had become too weak to move or even speak, yet the light in his eyes was still bright and he still smiled sweetly at me from time to time. He could also muster the strength to squeeze my hand occasionally and no other communication seemed necessary. The predominant sound and movement in those intimate moments was the breath moving in and out of his very frail body. After awhile, I noticed that R was holding his breath frequently, perhaps in resistance to some physical discomfort or in resistance to his rapidly approaching transition. I began to encourage him, both verbally and with gentle touch over his heart, to let his breath go rather than hold it. I thanked him each time he complied with the instruction. Every time I noticed him holding his breath I would whisper again, "Let the breath go," as I rested a hand on his chest or moved my hand ever so gently back and forth on his belly. He looked at me questioningly at one point and I said softly, "You're holding your breath." "Oh," he responded, smiling as if amused by the joke as he exhaled and we continued breathing together in silence.

AUTHOR

experiencing pain—physical, emotional or mental—and who is interested in meeting that pain with mercy, nonjudgment and love instead of with denial or fear.

We often try to lessen the sensations and emotions we label "pain" by pretending they don't exist, by ignoring them or by distracting ourselves in any and every way we can think of. Yet our resistance seems to increase rather than decrease our suffering. Often, simply putting our attention on our discomfort, fear or sadness and acknowledging its existence lessens its impact. Describing our experience and getting that experience across to someone else is also a way of alleviating pain.

You may support someone in bringing discomfort into conscious awareness through words as well as through your physical contact with that person. If the person you are working with is able to communicate verbally, you might ask him or her to describe the pain to you. Where is it located? How big is it? What color is it? Does the pain have a shape? Is it round, flat, rough, smooth, hot, cold? If you are working with people who are not verbal, simply ask them to notice these things.

As you observe, on a physical level, holding patterns in someone's body (muscles contracted around an area of discomfort or disease, for instance), ask that person to notice what thoughts arise in regard to the discomfort, or what feelings he or she might experience while holding the attention on that part of the body. The person may do this silently or may share his or her thoughts and feelings with you as you continue to guide this meditative exploration. You might ask a person to breathe into the pain, surround the pain with love, or to touch the pain with forgiveness. This kind of exercise in awareness can help an individual to detach, or de-identify, from intense emotional states. It can change the relationship of the individual to the pain that is being experienced, thus reducing anxiety and suffering.

Never force any technique or process on someone who is not open to receiving it or who does not express some interest in trying it. If you insist on using a technique with someone who is resistant to you or to the technique, not only will the potential benefits of the technique go unrealized, the relationship between you and that individual will be impaired.

SHARED BREATHING

Bringing your breath into harmony with the breathing pattern of another person is a simple way to create an alliance. Matching your breath to the breath of the person you are relating to during a touch session can give an even deeper dimension to your connection with that individual. You can use this technique at any time, whether the other person is asleep or awake. Sometimes it just happens spontaneously while you are massaging or bathing another or simply sitting quietly by the bedside of someone who is nearing death.

As a technique, shared breathing is accomplished by first becoming conscious of your own breathing as you inhale and exhale. The next step requires putting your attention on the breathing pattern of the other person. You can then begin to adjust the rhythm of your own breathing in order to synchronize your inhalation and exhalation of breath with the person whom you are observing.

When practiced at length, this experience of shared breathing can evolve into a surprisingly powerful exercise. It tends to heighten one's awareness of the breathing process and often creates a sense of calm or peace in both people. It may even produce a deep emotional catharsis for one or both individuals.

When someone is quite ill or near death, that person's breathing pattern can become irregular, in which case it becomes more difficult, though not impossible, to synchronize the breath. You may be able to help such a person stay conscious and aware in the moment by staying in contact with him or her and perhaps talking that person through each breath (much as you might support a woman going through a natural childbirth process.)

A great consolation can be given to the very ill simply by touching their hands, looking into their eyes, gently massaging them, or holding them in your arms, or breathing in the same rhythm gently with them.

SOGYLA RINPOCHE

Communication
Skills

ACTIVE LISTENING

Listening is a crucial component of relating to those in later life stages. People who are in crisis as well as those who feel isolated, alone or abandoned may need to talk, yet nobody has the time to hear what such people may need or want to say.

Most of us probably believe that we know how to listen. However, listening is much more than just waiting for our turn to talk. What I would call authentic and active listening is a communication skill that can be consciously developed and improved upon. It involves focusing one's attention, not just on what another person is saying, but on the individual who is talking. It means putting aside exterior and interior commentary in order to try to understand precisely what the person is expressing, listening not just to the words, but to the meaning behind the words and to the silences between words.

Active listening does not involve strain or effort. In fact, making an effort only gets in the way. The active listener simply puts his or her attention on the one who is communicating, patiently receiving the essence of whatever is being expressed without thought of any correct response.

The active listener

- is alert and present in the moment
- remains open to the other individual
- listens without evaluating or judging what is being said
- listens without interrupting, except to ask for clarification if necessary so that misunderstanding does not escalate

Perhaps true healing has more to do with listening and unconditional love than with trying to fix people.

GERALD JAMPOLSKY, M.D.

If only the doctors and nurses could realize that if they just took five minutes to listen to my mom—even though they can't do anything to change what is wrong with her—if they could just let her talk and listen, it would be like giving her a tablespoon of endorphins.

DAUGHTER OF FACILITY RESIDENT

Siddhartha listened. He was now listening intently, completely absorbed, quite empty, taking in everything... And all the voices, all the goals, all the yearnings, all the sorrows, all the pleasures, all the good and evil, all of them together was the world. All of them together was the stream of events, the music of life...

HERMANN HESSE, *SIDDHARTHA*

The ability to truly listen without interrupting or commenting, to receive and accept a communication without judgment is a valuable skill. When this ability is developed, it is, in and of itself, a significant and powerful healing technique.

I agree with Rachel Naomi Remen who says in *Kitchen Table Wisdom* that "Listening creates a holy silence. When you listen generously to people, they can hear truth in themselves, often for the first time. And in the silence of listening, you can know your self in everyone."[37]

Listening is one of the best therapeutic tools there is, when practiced skillfully. The very act of listening well can dissolve the distance we create between ourselves and others allowing words to disappear altogether so that two souls simply meet in a timeless moment, and awaken to the actuality of their connection.

POSITIVE INSTRUCTION

Positive instruction is a deceptively simply communication skill. It means that you tell someone what to do rather than what not to do. It is a good practice to follow in any relationship and it is especially effective as an aid in communicating with young children or with confused elders. This is because it is actually easier to follow or comply with a positive instruction. A negative instruction can subtly imply that someone has done something wrong or is being judged or evaluated, and tends to engage the mind at a deeper and more reactive level.

A friend of mine once saved her young son from a potentially dangerous situation on an boat trip because she knew he was used to following positive instructions. The excursion guide said several times, "Don't put your hand there" but the boy didn't respond until his mom intervened, calling him by name, and telling him, "Put your hands in your lap!"

Examples of positive versus negative instruction:

Positive Instruction	Negative Instruction
"Sit down here."	"Don't sit there."
"Keep your shirt on for now."	"Don't take your shirt off."

Reinforcing a positive instruction with guiding touch is especially helpful.

Just as most young children whose attention is engaged in another activity will not readily respond to a parent calling out some instruction such as "Okay, put all your toys away and come in and eat lunch," an elder coping with dementia or various physical frailties may have difficulty responding to multiple instructions. Experienced parents know that it is often necessary to go to the child, physically help that child put away the toys, take the child by the hand and lead him or her to the washroom, then to the table, then gently settle the child into the chair and push the chair to the table. Each step must be taken incrementally, and physical guidance given in order to produce the desired outcome.

Just as the child needs to be helped through each step and given support and acknowledgment as each step is completed, the frail elderly and the ill are often in need of such support and guidance as well. Both patience and persistence on the part of the person giving the instructions is called for.

ACKNOWLEDGMENT

Acknowledgment is another simple yet very powerful communication tool. It means letting a person know in some way that you have received his or her thought, that you have heard what was said and that you have understood what you heard. Acknowledgment should be genuine and never faked. In other words, if you did not understand something do not pretend that you did. Ask for clarification on anything that you did not understand before acknowledging.

You can acknowledge a communication with a simple "thank you" or "I understand" or "I get it" or through reflective or interpretive feedback as described on the following page. When someone follows an instruction you have given, you can acknowledge that compliance with some form of "thank you" or with a comment. Acknowledgment can be reinforced through eye contact, facial expression or conscious touch.

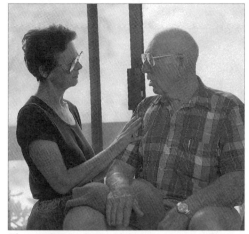

Photographer: James Patrick Dawson

Some people are hesitant to acknowledge a communication unless they agree with what the person is saying. It is not necessary to agree with what someone says in order to let the person know that you have received or understood his or her thought!

The universe is cluttered with incomplete communication cycles! When acknowledgment is repeatedly left out of the communication process, it generates unclarity, furthers misunderstanding and affects people in a variety of other ways. Some may conclude that it is useless to keep trying and give up communicating at all with certain people. Others may become angry with those whom they perceive as not "getting" their communications and engage in all sorts of strange, extreme and even self-destructive behavior in an effort to get their thoughts and feelings acknowledged.

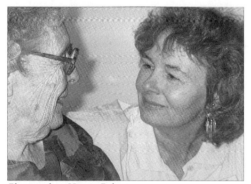

Photographer: Hunter Bahnson

As I was walking down the hall of the nursing home, I passed a woman alone in her room, sobbing softly. I knocked and walked into the room. Kneeling down beside her, I touched her gently on the arm. She blurted out between great sobs: "I just realized that we are going to be here for the rest of our lives. We're never going back to our home." I felt the emotional impact of that realization for her. I said, "I'm sorry. That must be really hard for you." This acknowledgment seemed to open the space for her next wave of emotion to surface. She told me that her husband was in another room and she didn't understand why they couldn't be together. It didn't seem fair to her that they should be in separate rooms. I agreed that it didn't seem fair and offered her my hand. She took hold of it and squeezed tightly. She then looked at me directly for the first time and said, "I just want to be able to reach out and touch him." I stayed with this woman for awhile, holding her hand, stroking her back and neck and just receiving her sadness. I wasn't certain if her husband was dead, at home, or actually in another room in the facility. I told her I would tell the unit manager that she was feeling sad and missing her husband. I did not say I could change anything or that the facility could change anything, just that I would pass the information on. The unit manager confirmed that this resident and her husband had both lived in the facility for almost five years, in separate rooms because that particular unit was not set up for two people to be in the same room. I was also told that she was sometimes wheeled down to her husband's room during lunch time and that her presence almost always seemed to agitate him. About a month later, apparently for financial reasons, these two residents were transferred to another floor in the same facility and put into a double room.

Author

You cannot truly listen to anyone and do anything else at the same time.

M. SCOTT PECK

When communication cycles are complete, relationships tend to flow more easily and smoothly. Acknowledgment plays an important part in effective communication with anyone and perhaps holds special significance when relating to the elderly and the ill.

REFLECTIVE FEEDBACK

I use the words *reflective feedback* to refer to a response that arises out of active listening. It reflects or mirrors back to the one who has been speaking, what you, as the listener, understood. The point is not to repeat the exact words that were spoken but to demonstrate your understanding of what was said by reflecting back to the communicator, in your own words, what you heard. Reflective feedback is an excellent way to avoid some of the misunderstandings and problems that arise in relating to others.

Example:

Communication: "I can't stand the food in this place."

Reflective Feedback: "You really don't like the food here!"

INTERPRETIVE FEEDBACK

This kind of feedback, or response, to a communication goes a step further than reflective feedback in that you, as the listener, interpret what the person has said before reflecting it back. For instance, a person may be complaining in a loud voice about his or her care in some way—"The food is never hot;" "They always keep me waiting;" "They make me take a bath…" If you were using reflective feedback, you might respond to the last outburst by saying, "You don't want to take a bath." Using interpretive feedback to respond, you might say, "It must be difficult to have so little control over your life."

The first response is an acknowledgment that you have received and understood what the person has expressed. The second response is an acknowledgment of something deeper that the person is trying to get across, an acknowledgment of what that person may be experiencing underneath the words which have been spoken. You are uncovering the subtext so to speak. By your interpretive feedback, you are actually giving that person an opening to access and express deeper feelings. You will usually know intuitively what the deeper communication is, if there is a deeper communication there.

When you are correct and you use this form of response, you will often notice an immediate change in the person with whom you are communicating. The person may begin sobbing or may begin to vent his or her frustration or anger. It is important to simply listen and receive whatever is being expressed, without judging it, analyzing it or trying to fix anything.

On more than one occasion, when I've been working with the seriously ill, a person has asked me to give him or her something to speed up the death process. Rather than begin a discussion on the philosophical, moral or legal implications of such a request, I have tried to acknowledge, not just what was said but the unexpressed thought beneath the spoken words. In the case of a gentleman who asked me if I could get him some hemlock, I responded by saying "Are you feeling like you want to die?" He answered in the affirmative and spoke at some length about the matter. This is another example of interpretive feedback.

In any case, try to avoid evaluating, judging or analyzing what a person says. Be prudent, also, about continually sharing your own experiences. Self-disclosure may occasionally be supportive and appropriate, but your own experience should be shared only if it would be truly helpful to the person you are serving. It is usually best to simply listen, with all your available senses, understand as well as you can, and receive what the person is expressing. You can check out your understanding through either reflective or interpretive feedback, when possible.

UNIQUE CHALLENGES

When relating to the elderly and the ill, communication can sometimes seem quite challenging. Many elderly people are hard of hearing. Some wear hearing aids. Several times I have been interacting with someone in a care facility who seemed to be having difficulty hearing only to discover that a hearing aid had been removed or turned off or that a battery was no longer working.

Stroke survivors may be suffering from aphasia resulting from damage to the communication centers of the brain, which creates problems for that person in understanding words or remembering particular words or in accessing or expressing words. A form of aphasia, known as paraphasia, a condition in which a person has lost the power to speak correctly, can be especially frustrating. Such a person substitutes one word for another or jumbles words and sentences in such a way as to make speech nearly unintelligible.

Imagine yourself in a world where you are unable to say the words you intend to speak or you cannot understand words being spoken to you. You try to say "house" and the word "book" comes out of your mouth or someone asks you if you are thirsty and you hear only garbled, nonsensical words! Some people assume that a person suffering from aphasia is mentally incompetent. The frustration of not being able to communicate accurately or well may make the person with the condition appear uncooperative and depressed.

Here are some additional suggestions for interacting with stroke survivors or others who have difficulty with verbal communication:

1. Make sure you have the person's attention before speaking and make eye contact, whenever it is possible to do so.

2. Focus on the kind of communication that works best (verbal or written).

3. Use short sentences, adding appropriate gestures as much as possible.

I was in a room in a care facility where three elderly ladies resided. My client was the lady in the bed closest to the hallway door. The resident on the opposite side of the room seemed to be sleeping. A thin, white-haired lady was sitting in a chair by the middle bed. She was fiddling with some large ear phones which rested on both her ears like earmuffs. She appeared to be trying to turn the volume up on the radio the earphones were attached to so she could hear better. The volume got louder and louder until it became quite distracting. I told the resident with whom I was doing the touch session that I would be right back and walked over to see if I could assist the lady with the headphones on, whom I assumed must be very hard of hearing. When I touched her gently on the shoulder and asked if I could help her, she replied that she couldn't hear "the durned music" and that something must be wrong with the radio. Upon closer inspection I saw that the headphones were turned so that the "speakers" were facing outward instead of in toward this resident's ears. She smiled gratefully when the situation was corrected and happily listened to her music throughout my session with the lady in the neighboring bed.

AUTHOR

I worked with one bedridden yet very alert and expressive woman who was Italian and spoke very little English. The first few times I visited this lady, I felt somewhat frustrated about this language barrier, and kept thinking I should learn some Italian so that we could communicate. Over the months, however, we developed a way of conversing that included a lot of facial and bodily expressions and gestures, and we had no trouble communicating our fondness for each other. When she was feeling especially good or pleased with something, she would break out into song from some Italian opera and when she was upset, she had no trouble expressing her displeasure.

AUTHOR

4. Slow down the speed at which you talk (it may take ten to fifteen seconds for the aphasic person to comprehend a key idea or concept).

5. Avoid pretending to understand something when you don't. Just try again later.

6. Never talk about the aphasic individual as if he or she is not present.

7. Avoid speaking for the person.

8. Understand that any recovery from aphasia is a journey fraught with fear, confusion, anger and anxiety.

You may find yourself in the position of helping care for someone who speaks a different language than you, for instance Spanish. If the person is commuicative and conversant, try to have someone who does speak Spanish explain to the person that you are not conversant in that language. Touch is a universal language and, as such, can be a useful communication resource in such situations.

When a person is unable to speak and yet he or she obviously wants to communicate something and is able to write, you can try using a dry erase board or writing pad to facilitate the communication. I knew a woman who was temporarily unable to speak after a surgical procedure, who carried on quite animated conversations in this way with her visitors.

If you are spending time with someone who seems unable to communicate at all, always tell the person who you are and why you are there. Even if a person is in a comatose state, explain from time to time what you are doing. People have been known to come out of comas or to recover from strokes and to remember everything that was said and done while they were unable to respond. *Be very conscious about asking someone something when that person is unable to answer. Make statements rather than asking questions!*

Guidelines and Suggestions for Touch Sessions

BEFORE THE TOUCH SESSION

If you are providing a service, on either a professional or volunteer basis, and are working with those in later life stages, it is wise to call a few hours before any scheduled appointment to confirm that you are coming. There may have been some significant change in the person's condition, including death, that would be important for you to know. An overwhelmed caregiver may have forgotten the appointment or gotten confused as to who was coming when. The patient or the resident may have been relocated and no one thought to get in touch with you. It is also important to inform those involved as soon as possible if you are unable to keep a scheduled appointment for any reason. Try to avoid any last minute disappointments for those you see on a regular basis.

Care facility residents as well as elders who live alone sometimes have very few visitors from the larger community. If you are helping care for or offering touch sessions to such a person, it is important to remember that you may well become a more important part of that person's life than he or she is in yours. If you skip a scheduled visit it may be very upsetting to that person. He or she may feel abandoned or may worry that something has happened to you.

The gift of life... is no less beautiful when it is accompanied by illness or weakness... mental or physical handicaps, loneliness or old age. Indeed, at these times, human life gains extra splendor as it requires our special care, concern, and reverence.

CARDINAL TERENCE COOKE

When someone who is not an employee comes into the facility from the outside world, that person's relationship with the resident sometimes takes on a special quality. As the trust builds and the relationship develops, the resident feels that she has a new friend. The resident may confide in that person or share concerns that have not been voiced to healthcare workers or to family members. A massage practitioner may find out something about a resident that we didn't know or something the resident never communicated before and this is helpful to our staff because they get to know our residents better and to provide better care for the whole person.

BRIANNA ALLEN,
CARE FACILITY DIRECTOR

A sweet and usually quiet lady I used to see for massage sessions twice a week became almost distraught if I was even five minutes late on the afternoons I was scheduled to visit her. If I was unavoidably detained with another client or held up in traffic on the way to see her, I would find her outside her room pacing up and down in the hallway, anxious about my well-being.

In another case, a client who tended to be nervous and easily upset often became agitated if I didn't show up in her room by a certain time on my twice a month visits to the long-term care facility where she resided. Since the drive from my home to this particular facility took close to one hour and traffic was often unpredictable, I tried to explain that I was unable to estimate my arrival time closely. I did assure her that she would be the first person I came to see each time. This was before the era of cell phones. However, if I happened to get a late start on a particular day or had reason to believe I might arrive later than usual, I made sure to call and have a staff member tell her that I was on my way and looking forward to seeing her. I later realized that I could ask that a portable phone be taken to her bedside so that I could deliver my message in person. Then, if she said later that she did not get the message, I could remind her of some key word in our conversation or something else that was said. Busy staff members can get distracted or preoccupied with some other more pressing duty and fail to deliver your message.

Avoid spending time in healthcare facilities for the elderly and the ill if you are ill yourself! That is to say, if you have a fever, flu, cold or if there is any possibility that you may have contagious disease, refrain from getting close to or touching a person who is already physically weak and vulnerable. For the infirm, catching the flu could be very serious or even fatal.

It is also better not to offer a touch session to someone if you are extremely fatigued or in an emotional crisis, because your physical and mental state will be felt on some level by the person receiving your touch. It will influence the session and could affect that individual adversely. If you are able to override your own state of mind by focusing your attention on the other person, then go ahead with the session; if you cannot, then it is better to reschedule your visit or appointment.

Do your best to maintain your own physical and emotional health so that you will be able to offer your touch to others when you are needed or your presence is requested. If someone seems within hours or minutes of death and requests your services, then, even if you are ill, you will have to use your own judgment as to how important your presence is to that person and whether or not you are able to be with him or her.

Avoid wearing heavily scented perfumes or lotions during your touch sessions. Dress simply and comfortably in clothing that will not hamper your relating or be a distraction. File your fingernails short enough so that they will not interfere with any fingertip touch techniques you may want to use. Remove bracelets and rings and put them in a safe place prior to beginning a session.

Before entering the home or the room of the person you will be touching, take a few moments to ground and center yourself. You don't have to do anything elaborate or visually weird in front of other people. You may want to meditate in your own room or home before going to a session. You may choose to sit quietly in your car for a few moments before going into someone's home, or to pause briefly outside the door of a hospital room before entering.

You may choose to use a calming and centering technique as simple as putting your attention on your own physicality and becoming aware of your connection to the ground beneath you. Shifting your awareness to your breath, without even doing anything to change it, is a powerful focusing device. It can be quite effective as a calming and centering technique. Once your attention is focused on your breath, find the place in your body that you experience as your center and breathe deeply from that place.

I hesitated outside the home of the first hospice patient to whom I was assigned as a volunteer and the prayer that arose in my mind was, "Please let me keep my heart open and my mouth shut." Sometimes, before approaching the person I will be relating to, I repeat a silent meditative thought or affirmation. Sometimes I just focus on my breathing for a few minutes or I put my attention on opening my heart to include whatever it is that I may be fearful of or not wanting to accept in regard to that particular situation or person.

When relating to the elderly and the ill, do your best to set aside any specific agenda or goals that you may have in mind for your touch session. Make a commitment to be present, just to be with the person, whatever may occur. Approaching another individual with the attitude that we have the training or the skills or the right answers to "help" him or her only gets in the way of real relationship.

I have noticed that using the word "they" to describe any group of people creates a distance between me and that group. By merely using the word, I am subtly holding myself separate from and superior to those particular others. Referring to someone as a "victim" of his or her disease and even labeling someone as "a patient" suggests an unequal or co-dependant relationship and, on a subtle level, can be distancing.

Sometimes we are given a specific role to play in someone's life or a particular responsibility to fulfill. We may be introduced in the context of performing a certain task or service. Whenever possible, however, I have found it liberating to take the approach of simply being open to each person as an individual, allowing the relationship between us to unfold naturally.

Something else you may want to before you begin a touch session is to energize and warm your hands before making physical contact with another. There are many ways to do this. In terms of warming, you could, of course, simply hold your hands in front of a heater or wear hand warmers for a few minutes but these methods are not always available or practical. You may want to try some of the following exercises and see which one works best for you in terms of bringing energy into your hands and warming them quickly.

The fundamental delusion of humanity is to suppose that I am here and you are out there.

YASUTANI ROSHI

Palm Rub

This is probably the easiest and most natural way to warm your hands. Open your hands out flat with just a little natural space between the fingers. Bring the palms of your hands together and begin to rub them quickly back and forth. Notice the heat that is generated as you do this. Increase the speed of your movements so that you feel even more heat and then let your hands relax.

Finger Flick

Make a small circle with each hand by curving your four fingers in toward the palm and bringing your thumb up to cover the nail of your middle finger. Pressing lightly on your middle finger with your thumb, free your fingers by quickly flicking them up and out from under your thumb. Do this with both hands at the same time, five times in quick succession, rest a moment and repeat.

A variation on this exercise is to simply squeeze both hands into fists and then flick the fingers and thumbs outward, spreading the fingers apart and opening the hands until you feel the skin on your palms stretching. You may feel a warm and tingly sensation in your hands after repeating this action a few times.

Handshake

Bring your arms up and slightly out to the sides with elbows bent. Let your wrists and hands be loose and shake your hands vigorously from side to side. Or, let your arms and hands relax at your sides and shake the whole arms from the shoulders so that you feel the shaking in your upper arms, lower arms and hands. Do this for about ten seconds, then relax. You may be aware of a tingling sensation, a warmth or a rush of energy in your hands and arms. Repeat the hand or whole arm shakes several times if you wish.

Fingernail Polish

Bring both hands up in front of you. Curl the fingers downward. Bring the fingernails of both hands to rest against each other. Holding one hand steady, move your other hand back and forth quickly as if you were polishing the fingernails of the other hand with a brush. Relax and repeat.

Visualization

Other exercises you can do to prepare your hands for touching someone (in addition to thorough hand washing of course) do not involve any movement at all. If you are good at visualizing, imagine a stream of warm light radiating out from your heart, down through your arms and into the palms of both hands. You can also try "breathing" into your hands by mentally following your breath as you exhale, directing it down your arms, into your hands and out through your fingertips. Sometimes it is helpful to make the light you are visualizing a specific color or imagine your breath being a specific color.

Mental preparation can also be helpful before you begin a touch session. Set aside any preconceived ideas you may have about the person you are about to touch and your opinions about his or her particular situation or condition. Take lightly any evaluative comments made by others concerning someone's personality or particular way of being. You may be told that a person you are about to see is always angry or uncooperative, or that a patient is in "heavy denial." However, your experience with that particular individual may be quite different from someone else's. This has happened to me numerous times. It is not necessary to invalidate your own experience or another person's perceptions, or to argue about the situation. However, if you relate to a person according to someone else's experience of that person's personality, or as if a written report about the person's condition is the absolute truth about him or her, then your relationships will lack reality in the present moment. Continue to approach each individual with an open mind and an open heart, each time that you come together, and let the session and your relationship unfold in its own way.

Being open means being willing to have things be however they are. Make a conscious decision to remain open during your touch session and to face whatever may occur. This will not always be an easy task. There may be times you will want to run away, break down sobbing, give up or give in to your own emotional reactions. These are natural impulses. You can note your reaction or your impulse and yet keep your attention on the individual you have chosen to relate to. This is another way of setting aside your own "stuff" in order to be present for and with another. This is not to say that you should never cry or let yourself be affected by what those you are working with may be experiencing. There will no doubt be times when you will feel emotionally affected by what occurs in your caregiving or touch sessions. You have a responsibility to be real and you should take the risk to be real even if that means letting your sadness show. Avoid dramatizing, however, or going into your own emotional reaction to the extent that the other person feels that he or she must comfort you. Notice what is coming up for you and avoid getting attached to your own emotions or shifting the attention to yourself. Keep your attention focused on the person you are working with. You might need to make a verbal acknowledgment to the person with whom you are working of what you are feeling in a particularly emotional moment. Doing so may help you let go of your own thoughts or emotions in order to bring your attention back to the person you are there to serve. Or, perhaps just making a mental note of what is coming up for you will be sufficient, knowing that you can process it more fully after your visit has ended.

Elders who are suffering from a dementia such as Alzheimer's and other kinds of age-related imbalances are likely to forget who you are from visit to visit. They may confuse you with someone else; they may even become inexplicably hostile and lash out at you in some way. It is possible to handle irrational outbursts and radical mood swings by simply ignoring the behavior and remaining focused on the individual. If someone you are working with should suddenly become aggressively angry or out of control, do not take it personally and do not allow yourself to be abused. Ask for help if you need it. Leave the room if you have to.

If you are a volunteer or professional practitioner offering massage sessions in home or facility settings, it may be helpful to procure some information from the nurse on duty, or from a primary caregiver regarding the physical condition of the person you are about to see,

Everybody has had a mother and a father and sooner or later we've got to treat our elderly clients the way we would our own parents.

WORKSHOP PARTICIPANT

before beginning a touch session. It is not necessary to know the person's entire medical history. However, in addition to the diagnosis, you might ask about recent changes in someone's physical or mental state or in prescribed medications. For instance, it would be helpful to know, if you are not already privy to such information, whether a person is taking a medication that is known to produce side effects such as itching, insomnia, depression, mood swings, headaches, and so on. It is also helpful to know if the person can stand or walk alone, and how much assistance he or she may need in turning in bed or in getting from one place to another. Remember that someone's mental and emotional state can greatly affect that person's physical condition and vice versa. Remember, too, that whatever condition or state a frail elderly or seriously ill person is in, it may shift or change very quickly.

As you enter the room or space where your touch session is to take place, take a few moments to assess the environment and make any minor adjustments that might facilitate a successful session. If you are seeing someone in a hospital or care facility who is in a room with more than one occupant, you will probably want to pull the curtain between the beds to allow for more privacy. If the person in the next bed is awake, you will want to acknowledge that person's presence in some way and reassure him or her that you will open the curtain before you leave.

You may need to move a small table or a chair to gain better access to the person you have come to see. If you are in a medical facility, do not move equipment such as oxygen tanks or IV stands without asking permission from the staff. Make sure to put anything you move back in its original place before you leave the room!

One thing I have learned in a decade of confronting the mechanics of hospital beds is that there are any number of different ways to raise and lower bedrails and to adjust the height of the bed itself. If you are at all in doubt, it is wise to check with a staff person to make sure it is all right to lower the guard rails on the bed. Remember to raise the rails again when the session is complete. *This is very important!* Put the bed height back to its original position, unless the person you are working with is able to do it or requests a different position.

You are, in essence, touching a person as soon as you enter the room where she or he occupies space. As you approach that person, remember that everything about you is touching him or her—your hands, your voice, your eyes, your facial expressions, and even your thoughts! Resolve to consciously give your undivided and focused attention to the person you have come to see or the person you are caring for during your touch session. Try to put your attention on him or her as an individual.

If you are a primary or relief caregiver offering touch to a patient or to a loved one, arrange to spend a certain amount of undistracted time with that person sharing this particular nurturing experience. Even though you may be touching your loved one as you attend to various tasks throughout the day, you can treat this time as special and focus your attention solely on her or him as you use specific touch therapy and other techniques that are not necessarily a part of more general physical care and treatment.

Protecting Yourself and the People You Touch

It is important to wash your hands *thoroughly* with soap and water before you begin a massage or touch session and again when you have completed the session. If you are professional practitioner seeing a number of people sequentially in a care facility, pay particular attention to this cleansing as you move from one resident to the next. In many facilities, you will find a sink with disinfectant soap in each room, or in an attached bathroom. If I am moving from room to room, after I see one person I go to the next person's room and wash my hands there before beginning the new session. On a subtle level this may help the person you are about to touch to feel protected, and it can avoid the possibility of making the last person you worked with feel that you find his or her body dirty or disgusting in some way.

Use common sense in avoiding direct contact with lesions, undiagnosed rashes or contagious skin problems. *Never* touch or massage directly on an open wound, weeping rash, laceration or bruise. You can work softly around or above such conditions and you might try laying a hand most gently on top of a bruise or healing fracture, simply letting your attention rest there, and letting the energy flow through your hands to that place.

In contagious situations, where direct physical contact with someone creates a health danger to either of you, it is possible to use some massage techniques or administer touch therapy wearing surgical gloves. These can be purchased in bulk at medical supply stores and should be discarded after each use. You can also use attentive touch techniques working over a sheet or thin blanket which acts as a shield between your hands and the body you are touching. Skin-on-skin contact is preferable, yet being touched through gloves or over covers is certainly better than being deprived of touch. Many touch techniques are still effective and most of the benefits remain the same.

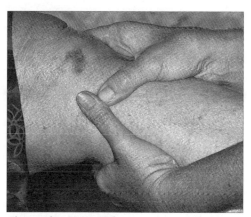

Photographer: Hunter Bahnson

You may occasionally need to work on top of, or reach underneath, bed covers, or even clothing, to administer massage to an older person who chills easily. I used to visit a ninety-eight-year-old gentleman who walked on his own and could still bend over and tie his own shoes every morning. However, he was thin, his movement was limited and he chilled easily. This man usually wore a woolen hat, neck scarf and gloves over his clothing no matter what the weather. He often had on several layers of clothing even when he was in bed underneath the covers! He sometimes wanted to take off an outer jacket for his back rub and I would simply work over the rest of his clothing.

Protecting yourself energetically or psychically can be advantageous before beginning a touch session. This may sound mystical but it is actually quite practical. Some people easily "take on" or absorb another person's physical or emotional state of being without even realizing it. I learned very early on in my massage practice that if I did not consciously guard against it, I would frequently experience whatever symptoms my client was manifesting by the end of our hour together! This included physical complaints such as stomach and headaches as well as emotional states such as anxiety or depression.

There are various ways to solve this problem. The grounding and centering exercises suggested earlier will help. You can visualize yourself surrounded by a golden or white light or protected inside an invisible bubble or band of energy. You can repeat a short affirmation or prayer of protection. Or, you can simply make a conscious decision before you begin a touch session not to take on that person's physical symptoms, emotional feelings or mental attitudes.

One aspect of taking care of yourself is to insure your own comfort during your touch sessions. By taking the time to do this, you will avoid unnecessary pain and fatigue, and you will be able to continue giving your energy and full attention to the person you are touching. If you are standing, be sure to keep your knees slightly bent rather than "locked." Bring a hospital bed up to a workable height, if possible, so that you don't have to bend over, or figure out a way to sit down while you work. Use a knee pad or rolled-up towel to protect your knees when kneeling beside a person in a wheelchair and remember to keep breathing!

During my initial visit to one chronically ill gentleman, I put my own body in various awkward positions in order to reach him when it was completely unnecessary to do so. I was simply too self-conscious to ask questions concerning his mobility or even to ask for a chair to sit on. I stood for awhile working over the bed rails when they didn't release easily, and eventually I got on my knees and reached between the bars. I stretched my upper body over a table that could have been moved and generally made things difficult for myself in any number of ways. I was physically exhausted after I left and needed a massage to recover! I have never repeated that particular mistake!

DURING THE TOUCH SESSION

Be cognizant of the physical limitations of the person with whom you are working. Some infirm people are able to walk slowly by themselves or with help, and may prefer to see you while sitting in a favorite chair (a recliner chair works quite well if one is available) or lying on a sofa. Many people you work with will be confined to a bed or a wheelchair. Some will be able to sit up or turn over and some will not. Again, adapting yourself and the techniques you use to the situation as you find it is the key!

Pain is frequently communicated through nonverbal behavior. In working with those in later life stages, you must learn to look for these nonverbal indicators of discomfort. One good way of assessing discomfort is to watch the breathing pattern of the patient. Someone who is acutely stressed, anxious or in pain will usually exhibit irregular breathing. A person may seem to hold his or her breath at intervals or take very long and deep breaths. He or she may breath so shallowly that it is difficult to tell whether or not breathing is occurring at all. A person may breathe very rapidly and deeply, almost to the point of hyperventilating. As a person relaxes you will notice the breathing pattern becoming more normal. Someone may switch from chest to abdominal breathing. Another person may yawn or let out a long sigh after which the inhalation and exhalation of breath will become more regular and even.

I have more medicine than a pharmacy. I now take forty-five pills a day. It's a bit ridiculous but it seems to get the job done.

FROM A CANCER PATIENT'S JOURNAL

In relating to the elderly and the ill, it is important to develop your powers of observation and to train yourself to pick up on cues as to what kind of pain is being experienced and where it may be coming from. The person you are touching may not be able to answer the question "Does it hurt here?" or "Is this area tender?" and so you must rely on what your hands can feel, your observation of subtle nuances or changes in a person's body or behavior, and your intuition.

Do not be surprised at any sudden change in the desires or the requests of the aged and the ill. Remember, too, that minds may be less agile and more forgetful during the aging process and that medications can add to disorientation and mental confusion.

A seriously ill person may become too weak or too uncomfortable to speak, or may wish to talk only with certain people. Occasionally a family member or another care provider will tell you that someone is unable to talk or is verbally incoherent, yet during the time you are with him or her, that person will speak in perfectly understandable words. You must use your best intuitive sense in deciding whether or not to tell the person from whom you received the original communication about such an occurrence. It is possible that the ill person has something to communicate and simply cannot say it to a loved one, or senses that a family member is not ready to hear it. That family member may feel hurt that the patient or loved one talks to you and yet remains silent around her or him, and may then become angry and aloof toward the patient or, more likely, toward you. Try to ascertain the effect it could have to pass information which you are given along to someone else and whether or not it would actually be helpful to do so before you make a decision. Always encourage family members to keep talking to their loved ones even if the loved one does not reply or seems not to hear.

I remember sitting with a woman who had been doing battle with cancer for a long time. She'd gone through surgery, chemotherapy and radiation treatments and had eventually been told by her doctors that nothing more could be done to arrest the progression of her disease. The second time I visited her in her home she was very still and quiet. We were alone in her bedroom together and at one point she seemed to summon up all her energy in order to speak. She said that she just didn't see how she could do anything more. She nodded when I acknowledged that she must be very tired. I understood her to mean that she had done all she could to stay alive and that she was ready to die. It seemed as if she simply needed to communicate this to someone. Perhaps it was easier for her to say those words to me, a relative stranger, than to her husband or her adult children. Though her family seemed prepared to let her go, I suspect it was easier for me to tell her that she needn't do anything more, that she could rest. Without making any more attempts to speak to anyone, this lady died peacefully in her sleep a day or two later.

V's daughter, who was exhausted, hired me to care for her mother. I took care of V three evenings a week from 8 p.m. to 7 a.m. for three weeks. She was in the later stages of Alzheimer's disease and was dying from breast cancer. She was confused most of the time and in terrible pain. She knew something wasn't right and it frightened her. When I was hired, her daughter whispered to me in confidence, "She is dying, she doesn't know and we don't want her to know." This was difficult for me. I felt stuck between honoring the family's wishes and respecting V's process. One evening before bedtime, she asked, "Am I going to die?" Those very words were the clearest and most profound she had spoken the entire time. I responded by saying "What I know is that you are very, very sick." She seemed to understand my words and those I could not speak. The following week, I arrived to find her in a worse condition. That evening, I was awakened by her moaning. I came into her room and quietly sat beside her. Within minutes, she bolted up out of bed and very forcefully and distinctly uttered the words, "Bye! Bye!" She even waved goodbye. Then she collapsed into her bed and slipped into a coma. I sat with V and held her hand throughout the night. She died peacefully the next morning. There is a place of knowingness amidst the confusion within all of us.

SHOSHONA FRIEDEN, L.M.T.

POSITIVE AND NEGATIVE INDICATORS

I once worked with a woman in a convalescent home twice a week for nearly a year. This woman, who had suffered a stroke shortly before I began seeing her, was not able to speak and, in fact, she sometimes slept through our sessions. At other times, however, she would reach for my hand or look at me directly for long periods of time. Occasionally, she made some sounds as if trying to speak. I took this as a positive indicator and always acknowledged it as such.

In this type of situation you must learn to watch for and feel subtle signs of response and relaxation. Indications that person is responding to your attention and touch in a positive way could include

- body relaxation (i.e. shoulders dropping, head dropping forward, hands opening, arms or legs uncrossing, the mouth opening)
- tight muscles softening or releasing
- sounded release such as a groan, or "purr"
- breath release or sigh
- change in breathing pattern from chest to belly, fast to slow or irregular to regular
- any movement toward you
- eyelids flickering or opening
- person making eye contact
- a genuine smile
- release of gas or odor from body
- stomach "gurgling"
- a change in skin color (from white to pink)
- a change in body temperature (from cold to warm)
- emotional release or expression such as sadness, anger, sobbing
- yawning
- falling asleep, snoring
- increased consciousness of body parts or sensations in body
- verbal affirmation

Negative indicators or signs that a person is not responding well to your attention or your touch could include

- holding or tightening of body parts
- clenching fists or crossing arms
- stiffening of head or neck
- clenching of teeth or jaw
- holding breath
- change in breathing pattern from belly to chest, slow to fast, or regular to irregular
- frown or facial grimace
- a gruff sounding snarl or "growl"
- movement away from you
- physical agitation
- continued body rigidity
- body jerking or twitching
- verbal insults

Sometimes it is difficult to "read" the clues or the behaviors you are observing. In fact some indicators might be interpreted as positive or negative, depending on the circumstances and upon what else is occurring at the time These could include

- giggling
- crying
- rapid talking
- no visible or verbal response at all

MEDICAL EQUIPMENT AND APPARATUS

If you are relating to people in skilled nursing facilities or to those living at home with the help of hospice, you will at some point find yourself having to work around or deal with various kinds of medical machinery and equipment such as

- feeding tubes
- catheters
- Intravenous lines
- oxygen tanks and tubes
- aspirators
- monitors

Most such devices will actually be attached to the person you are caring for. When you are unfamiliar with it, such paraphernalia can be distracting, even frightening. If you do not have direct experience in handling such objects, it is helpful to educate yourself as to their functions since the person you are relating to may be dependent upon them. You must be very careful as you move around a bed, for example, not to stand on tubing that might cut off oxygen or to accidentally pull or step on catheter tubing, which could cause acute discomfort for the person using the tube.

This is another area in which your creativity and flexibility will be helpful. You will need to adapt whatever massage or touch techniques you are using and invent new ways of working as you go along. There is almost always more than one way to accomplish a task. (It also helps to have a sense of humor!)

If you are lotioning or massaging large areas of a person's body, you may encounter diapers, bandages, dressings, narcotic patches, and so on. If you are using long strokes on the legs or thighs, you may want to unfasten the side of a diaper in order to massage the buttocks. Always ask permission of the person whose body you are touching, if he or she is able to respond, before doing this. Proceed non-intrusively and with respect for the person's dignity and privacy at all times.

Loss of control over one's life, on many different levels, is usually a major issue for a rapidly aging or seriously ill person. A person in such a situation must submit to all kinds of intrusive, uncomfortable, undignified and even embarrassing procedures in the course of diagnosis and treatment of a life-threatening illness. Nearly everyone experiences some loss of privacy and individuality during a stay in a medical facility. In such places, numerous rules, regulations and procedures are carried out according to a strict time schedule which is based on keeping a large institution functioning smoothly, rather than

We never lost our sense of humor!

PRIMARY CAREGIVER AFTER DEATH OF
FAMILY MEMBER

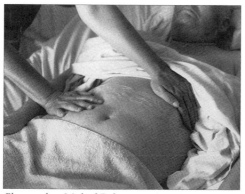

Photographer: Michael Pedersen

Every time I asked the gentleman I was doing the touch session with a question, his wife, who was usually sitting on the other side of the room knitting during my visit, answered for him. This man was not particularly talkative during our session, though he did occasionally initiate a conversation with me, and he always answered me when his wife was out of the room; so it seemed that the wife's speaking for her husband was just part of the dynamic of their relationship. Sometimes I rephrased the question slightly and, after making sure I really had this gentleman's attention, I would ask again, giving him a chance to answer me directly. Eventually we developed a kind of shorthand in which I would ask the question, his wife would answer, I would look at him, and he'd smile and then nod either yes or no. I also noticed that when I assured his wife that I would give her a back rub too before leaving, she began to busy herself with other things during my session with her husband, which gave him more autonomy in our interaction.

AUTHOR

on the individual preferences, desires or wishes. A person's professional position, status or social standing in the outside world matters little inside the hospital room.

As already noted, residents of nursing homes and extended care centers are required to follow someone else's schedule in most matters. Their choices are greatly limited and they often have little privacy. I have observed men and women in such facilities struggling to maintain their dignity as they experience what appears to be their personal power slowly slipping away. One of the most compassionate things you can do for people in such circumstances is to give them as much autonomy and control as possible during the time you spend with them. Let the nursing home resident or the person occupying the hospital bed know that during your interaction, he or she is "the boss." Ask the elderly for permission to call them by their first names, sit on their beds, or to move personal articles.

Avoid the temptation to do things for others that they may be able to do for themselves. Ask a person if he or she needs help getting into bed or getting a glass of water instead of assuming that help is needed. Direct your questions and comments to the person with whom you are doing the touch session (rather than to the caregivers or family members) if that person is capable of responding.

Honor the choices of your loved ones, friends and clients whenever possible. Let each person set the tone for your touch sessions or your time together. If a person is able to communicate well, allow her or him to lead the conversation and talk about whatever may be important. Give an opinion only if you are asked directly and refrain from lengthy "sharing" of your own experiences and points of view. Ask simple questions that will encourage the person to expand on what she or he is telling you. Then be quiet and listen!

If a person is unable to communicate well with words, or simply tires of talking, make sure that you do not insist on a conversation or on answers to your questions. Let the person know that it is not necessary to talk, that you are happy to just sit with him or her or to continue your touch session in silence.

SEXUAL ENERGY

It is possible that, at some point, while you are administering massage or touching someone in a gentle, caring way, that person will become sexually aroused. This energy often manifests itself more obviously in men, yet it occurs in females as well. This is a natural and understandable response, especially when you are working with people who may have been deprived of gentle, nurturing touch for an extended period of time. You need not judge or negate the person's experience. On the other hand, you must be very clear about your own intentions and boundaries in your relationship with those whom you touch.

I was once giving complimentary mini-massages at a health fair being held in a multi-level care facility. A student colleague of mine was working alongside me. She was on her knees touching an elderly gentleman's legs when he said that he was experiencing discomfort in his knees. She rolled up his pant legs and began massaging around his knees all the while continuing to chat with him. I noticed that the minute she touched an area just above his knees his conversation began to take on subtle sexual overtones and then I head him say "I have a vibrator." My colleague was completely unaware of this connection. She had been distracted and taken her attention off what she was doing or what he was saying in that moment.

It may be necessary to verbalize restrictions regarding sexual boundaries to someone who is confused. If the person is mentally alert and able to speak, you can address the issue of sexual energy directly. You can acknowledge the deprivation that the person must be feeling, letting him or her know that the feelings are okay and acceptable, and that you understand how frustrating it must be to be unable to act on those impulses. Your acknowledgment, acceptance and understanding will go far toward alleviating that frustration and helping the person to feel satisfied by the contact you can offer.

I have learned through experience to be open to the unexpected when working with people who are mentally distracted and disoriented. It is good to remember that age, discomfort, medications and loneliness can evoke behavior in people that is not always appropriate or rational.

One day I began giving a foot massage to a gentleman I had seen previously a few times, as he lay dozing on his bed. This man was close to ninety, blind and not always totally coherent. A few minutes into the session, the man unzipped his pants, exposed himself and began to engage in an activity not normally conducted in front of others. When he did not respond to my suggestion to zip his pants or to turn over, I covered him with a light blanket. I told him that he obviously needed some privacy and that I would be back to see him the following week.

In reflecting on this incident, I realized that I could have avoided this somewhat awkward situation. In subsequent visits, if I found this gentleman in bed, I made sure to wake him up and talk with him for a few minutes before beginning the massage session. The problem never occurred again.

I have also learned not to use the phrase "What would you like?" or "What can I do for you?" unless I know a person very well. This type of open-ended question can occasionally create a challenging situation. I once had a kind-looking elderly gentleman in a wheelchair pull me down on his lap when I asked what I could do for him that day and proceed to tell me in very specific language what he wanted. I managed to extricate myself quickly from this startling incident and treated it with humor rather than embarrassment or outrage. After a similar situation occurred on another occasion with someone else, I learned to phrase the question differently.

Respect the individuality of each person you come in contact with. Put aside images or ideas you may have about how people should behave when they are seriously ill or nearing the end of their life's journey. Put aside your mental pictures of how you would want one of your loved ones to behave or how you think you might act in a similar situation. Remain open to each individual as you encounter him or her and to each experience as it unfolds. Do your best to accept whatever occurs and carry on.

We meet ourselves time and again in a thousand disguises on the path of life.

CARL JUNG

SYMPATHY, EMPATHY, COMPASSION

If you have a tendency to think of yourself as a "savior," you will have no trouble connecting with people who consider themselves "victims." These two types of personalities seem to attract each other like magnets. Many marriages and other relationships are held together by an unspoken agreement between two people to support one another in playing out these roles in life.

The nursing home population is no different from the world in general. Some people tend to constantly dramatize their "stories" and some are constantly complaining or feel victimized by their life dramas. Putting yourself into the middle of someone else's drama (ranting and raving against the unfairness of it all or joining in blaming and judgment) is not ultimately supportive if what you want is to serve the *individual*, who is something other than the drama, the story, or the role he or she may be presenting. What the person most needs is your authentic contact with who he or she actually is.

Over the years I have contemplated what it means to be sympathetic and what it means to feel empathy for another in the context of relating to the elderly, the ill and the dying. Imagine that you come upon a person who has fallen into a pit too deep to climb out of. How do you respond? What action can you take? It seems to me that the following definitions, though different from meanings found in most dictionaries, are applicable and that the distinctions are useful in this context.

- **Sympathy:** Kneel at the edge of the pit and tell the person how sorry or concerned you are.

- **Empathy:** Jump into the pit with the person.

- **Compassion:** Find or make a rope, throw it down to the person and either hold it or secure it to something so the person can pull him or herself out of the pit; if necessary, lower yourself into the pit, put the person on your back and climb back out.

EFFECTS OF CHANGING ENVIRONMENT

I have sometimes given touch sessions over a period of time to people in their homes and then visited those same people in a hospital or nursing home (or vice versa). The environment of a medical center or convalescent facility is quite different from the home environment and, naturally, certain adjustments must be made. In a medical setting, the surroundings are unfamiliar and the schedule is arranged for the convenience of the staff who are managing care for a group rather than for an individual.

You may observe noticeable changes in a person's behavior or attitudes when he or she is shifted to a new environment. The move itself may have been painful or otherwise traumatic. Certain things may seem easier or more difficult in one environment or the other. Family members may have varied positive or negative reactions to the change in location as well. Avoid getting caught in the middle of family conflicts. Remain positive in your interactions with all the people involved. Give your opinion only if specifically requested to do so. Remember that you can acknowledge a communication without agreeing with it. Never invalidate someone's personal experience or feelings.

In relating to those in later life stages, you may be seeing people who have no relatives or close friends, or those whose loved ones are too far away to visit often. In some cases, you may be, in effect, acting as a surrogate for those missing family members or close friends. Try to minister to those whom you touch as sensitively and care-fully as you would want someone to treat you or someone you love in a similar situation.

ENDING THE SESSION

Ideally, a touch session is open-ended in terms of time and is over when both you and the person you are working with feel satisfied that the session is complete. You might spend ten minutes with the person or you might spend an hour or even longer. Much of the time, however, and for various reasons, whether you are a professional practitioner, a volunteer or a family caregiver, your time will likely be limited to some extent; and so it is important to pace yourself and to set certain guidelines.

When you begin a touch session, whether you are offering your services on a volunteer or on a paid basis, if you have contracted for a specific amount of time or your timetable is limited, let the person you have come to see know how long the session will be or about how much time you have to stay with him or her. If you have the flexibility to stay longer, you can offer that option and give the person a choice. If you are charging a fee for services, you need to be clear in your own mind as to whether you are offering to extend the session on a volunteer or on a paid basis. If you are ambivalent about this, it will introduce unclarity and confusion into the relationship and it will affect your relationship with the other person.

I once heard a story about an experiment carried out in a large medical institution, in which a doctor went from room to room visiting with patients. Shortly after the doctor left the room, each patient was asked, "How long did the doctor spend with you?" The patients all said that the doctor had spent at least fifteen minutes, maybe more, in their rooms. In actuality, for the sake of the experiment, this doctor had spent exactly five minutes with each person. It was concluded that the patients felt the doctor had spent much longer with them than he actually had because in each instance

- he pulled up a chair and sat down beside the person
- he made eye contact with the person
- he held the person's hand during his stay

In other words, this doctor positioned himself so that he and the patient were at the same eye level and he gave each person focused physical contact! If you are able to be fully present during a touch session, giving the person your undivided attention, in my experience, that person will seldom be left wanting you to stay longer or to extend the session when it is time for you to leave.

I just come to work every day and I try to give them a little cheer. I treat these ladies like they was my grandmother.

AIDE IN ALZHEIMER'S FACILITY

If you are seeing someone whom you experience as being particularly "needy," you will have to be very clear about your own boundaries and, at the same time, be conscious about not judging the other person or making him or her wrong in some way. I have met people who were so desperate for attention that it seemed as if no amount of contact and acknowledgment would be enough. No matter how long I stayed, it was not long enough.

When I have a schedule to keep, and I know that a person may want me to stay longer than I am able, I often remind him or her at the beginning of the session how long I will be there. When the time allotted for the touch session is nearing an end, I give the person some warning, reminding him or her that I have a few more minutes to stay, and if possible, I find out what that person would like from me in those remaining minutes. I say something like "I have a few more minutes to be with you today. Would you like a short back rub before I go?" or "Shall I put a little lotion on your hands before I have to leave today?"

I usually carry a few objects with me (heart-shaped rubber "balls," small stuffed animals or extra finger puppets, a pretty handkerchief, and so on) that I am willing to part with if necessary. If a person is having difficulty with my leaving or is reluctant to let go of my hand, I leave something behind to occupy the person's hands and to ease my departure. Only once have I actually had to pry someone's hand open to extract my own at the end of a session. This man was nonverbal, and in an almost semi-comatose state, yet he always responded to my presence and my touch in some way. On this particular day he held onto my hand in a grip much stronger than I would have believed possible!

A student in one of my workshops ran into this problem once with an elderly resident in a skilled nursing facility. She had no objects to leave but solved the problem, I thought, in a most creative way. She said, "I've so enjoyed being with you today and I'm going to leave something for you to help you remember our visit." Then she kissed her

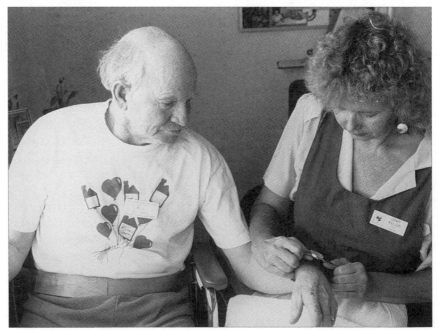

Photographer: Brock Palmer

hand and dropped the "kiss" into the lady's pocket as she and the resident exchanged big smiles and waved goodbye.

Remember to restore the environment to the way it was when you came into the person's personal space. (If you feel there is a very good reason for changing something, ask the resident of the room before doing so.) Put stockings and slippers that you may have removed back on the person's feet. If you have taken off someone's watch, remember to replace it. Be sure that you put the watch back on the same arm and in the same position in which you found it. I once noticed that I had put a gentleman's watch back on his arm in the reverse direction so that the face of his watch was upside down and not easily readable. This may seem like a little thing to us, but it can be quite frustrating to someone who has been partially paralyzed by a stroke or who has barely enough strength to lift an arm. It is particularly important to put bed trays back in the same position so that familiar and needed items may be easily reached.

It is very important that you raise the rails of the hospital bed before leaving, if that is the way they were when you arrived. If a resident asks you to leave the rails down, tell that person you are sorry but you are not allowed to do that. You can put the bed rail back the way it was and tell the resident you will let a staff person know that he or she wants it down. If you were to leave a bed rail down and the patient subsequently fell out of bed and was hurt, not only would you have to deal with your own feelings of responsibility in the matter, but both you and the facility could be found negligent in a lawsuit!

If you have been working with someone in a wheelchair, ask where he or she would like to be positioned before you leave. You might need to push that person back to a recreation area, for instance, or to a dining hall. If the person you have been visiting is communicative, tell that person that you are locking the wheels on her or his chair in place, unless you know that he or she is able to move the chair without help. When working with residents of convalescent or extended care facilities, never remove the safety belt on a wheelchair or try to help someone move from a chair into a bed or vice versa! If someone makes such a request, explain that you are not on the staff of the facility and you are not authorized to do such things but that you will relay his or her request to a staff member.

Caring for the Caregiver

CAREGIVER STRESS

If, as a volunteer or a paid service provider, you are seeing a chronically or acutely ill person in his or her home, be cognizant of the stress level of the family member or close friend who is acting as primary caregiver. Whether a person has consciously chosen to take on the responsibility of caring for a loved one at home or has simply fallen into the situation for financial or other reasons, he or she has taken on an enormous physical and emotional task. Being physically responsible for another adult is hard and fatiguing work; and it is painfully difficult to watch someone you love decline in health and strength.

There may be other loved ones acting as secondary or relief caregivers who are also under stress, and the relationships between these family members and caregivers may be strained. You might find yourself in the middle of a highly stressed family trying to cope with their own and others' reactions to a situation everyone wishes didn't exist. The family members will be in different stages of acceptance of their loved one's condition and they each may have different coping mechanisms. Try not to get caught in the middle of family discussions or disagreements or to get seduced into "taking sides." It is essential, both from a professional and a personal point of view, to remain impartial in such situations, and to give one's honest opinion, in a non-evaluative way, only if asked. Do not try to practice family therapy or counseling unless you are qualified to do so and unless your skills in that area are specifically requested.

I once drove to an address I'd been given to administer a touch session to a hospice patient for the first time. There was no response to the doorbell or to my gentle but persistent knocks on the apartment door. Just as I was turning to leave, a neighbor opened her door to tell me that the family had gone to the hospital a few hours earlier. I drove to the hospital, and found the patient's wife and son sitting outside one of the rooms on the hospice in-patient unit. I explained who I was and the patient's wife encouraged me to go see her husband. I found him, still alive but obviously near death, stretched out in a corpse-like pose on the hospital bed, a white sheet covering his legs, his hands folded atop his chest. The room was darkened and peaceful. I stayed with the man for awhile, touching him gently, letting him know that his wife and son were nearby and wishing him well on the next step of his journey. When I rejoined his wife and son, little was said beyond an acknowledgment of the reality of the moment. The woman readily accepted a back massage when I offered it. Her teenage son managed a polite smile when I introduced myself and then continued staring in stone-faced silence out the window. He seemed lost in a quiet desperate longing to be anywhere other than sitting outside that hospital room, to be doing anything other than waiting for his father to die. At his mother's urging, and perhaps to please her, he somewhat shyly agreed to let me touch him. As I gently massaged his back, I sensed his mind returning to his body from wherever his grief had taken him. His hunched up shoulders dropped as he began to relax and, eventually, to talk a bit.

AUTHOR

Caregivers frequently find themselves on an emotional roller coaster, experiencing a variety of feelings including fear, anger, frustration, abandonment, grief and loneliness, as well as love and compassion—all in the space of one long day! Those who have taken on the challenging responsibility of caring for an aging relative or a seriously ill loved one may, on any given day, be distressed, confused, irritable, depressed, overwhelmed and exhausted. They may not be able to afford to hire outside help or may be reluctant to do so for other reasons.

Caregivers often complain of physical pain in the neck and shoulders or back pain. This may be due to the strain of too much or improper lifting of an increasingly immobile person. It may also be a way of telling others that the burden is becoming too great, the load is too heavy to carry, and that some relief is needed. In other words, the pain, whether caused by physical misuse of the body or by mental or emotional anxiety and stress, is a warning signal and a cry for help.

You can support caregivers in various ways, in addition to offering them a back and neck rub or some other kind of massage. A simple acknowledgment of the reality of a situation can be enormously validating for a caregiver and may be deeply appreciated. If you mentally put yourself in a caregiver's shoes for a moment, it is easy to appreciate the labor and the courage of such a person, and to honestly comment on it. Avoid saying that you understand or know how the person feels unless you yourself have actually been in the exact same situation.

If the caregiver is open to it, a gentle squeeze of the hand, an arm around the shoulder or a touch on the heart can let the person know that you see the difficulty of the situation, that you sense his or her fatigue and level of stress. I sometimes ask caregivers what they do to nurture themselves. I encourage such people to take some time while I am working with their loved one, to take a walk or a shower, to do something refreshing or different, just for themselves.

I have observed that those caring for loved ones nearing death are sometimes reluctant to relax because they spend so much time trying to "hold things together," often denying their own needs and feelings in order to be there for the other person. These full-time caregivers may be afraid to relax even a little bit fearing that if they do they will fall apart completely and not be able to carry on. They may sense that letting themselves be nurtured and cared for will make them feel vulnerable or bring up feelings they are reluctant to face or accept. It is important to acknowledge and accept such fears or reluctance and not to challenge someone to move beyond what that person feels capable of in any given moment. At the same time, a gentle reminder to encourage caregivers not to let their own needs go unmet for too long or to push themselves too hard without relief is sometimes well received. Primary caregivers may be most in need, and more willing to accept massage or touch therapy in the weeks and months following the death of the loved one they are caring for. This is also the time when they may need emotional support more than ever.

One of the greatest gifts you can offer to an emotionally drained and weary caregiver is to simply listen and understand how it is for that person without imposing your own experience or opinions. Giving an individual your undivided and conscious attention for just five minutes, listening with your heart as well as with your ears, can have a greater impact than you might imagine.

SELF-CARE

"Take as good care of yourself as you do of patients," exhorts one nurse-thanatologist. It is essential for caregivers of all types to give the same kind of conscious attention to their own well-being that they do to those whom they serve or care for. I know many professional and even volunteer caregivers who fail miserably on this point. Why is it so difficult for us to comfort, nurture and cherish ourselves?

Taking care of yourself guards against caregiver stress and burn-out. Self-care includes setting limits, taking time to relax, and keeping yourself in balance physically, emotionally and mentally. It means treating yourself with the same mercy, loving-kindness, forgiveness and compassion that you offer your clients or those you are helping care for.

You cannot be all things to all people all the time. There are an endless number of people in the world who would no doubt benefit from being seen and listened to and touched. However, even if you decide to minister to such people as a full-time job or spend all your spare time as a volunteer in hospitals and care homes for the elderly, you will be able to connect with a relatively small number of those individuals. If you ignore your own needs, you will be able to work less and less productively with fewer and fewer people.

Working with people who are in crisis, who are in a great deal of pain, or who are experiencing a high level of stress and anxiety takes energy. It requires concentration. It forces us to focus our attention and open our hearts. It challenges us to push through our barriers and limitations, and sometimes, to go beyond what we think we are capable of, in order to remain present with a fellow human being who is being pushed way beyond what he or she ever thought possible or acceptable. It requires meeting our own pain with mercy as well as greeting the pain and suffering of others with mercy. If we are to be effective in serving others, we must allow our self-compassion to surface.

Watch for clues that will alert you to an imbalance in your life. If you are becoming irritable with or critical of your close friends and family members, if you are catching every flu and cold that comes around, if you are always tired, if you are overindulging in unhealthy substances, eating constantly or forgetting to eat, unable to sleep or sleeping more than usual, then it is probably time to stop, step back, and pay attention to what is really going on. You may want to lighten your load a bit or make a conscious effort to spend some extra time relaxing by yourself. You may need to take some time off to play with your family or close friends.

It is vital that you take whatever time and steps are necessary to make sure you continue to "refuel your own pump," so to speak. Just as we need to reduce, reuse and recycle our natural resources we need to relax, renew and regenerate our own energy so that we do not deplete

My father hired a caregiver nurse for six hours a day. We were fortunate that he had the resources to do this. The caregiver washed my mother daily and changed the sheets and did the wash. The rest of the time, night and day, either my sister or my father or I were with her, on a schedule we worked out. The dining room was converted into a room for my mother and she lay there on a hospital bed my father had rented. It was a pleasant room with lots of natural light and Mom could look out the windows at familiar sights. Friends could come and go easily and there was room for the the medical equipment that was eventually needed. At night I usually slept on a mat next to her bed. There was a button she could push which sounded an electronic bell in my father's bedroom upstairs. I saw fairly early how the phenomenon of caregiver fatigue could easily have closed in on us if these practical elements hadn't been set up.

LAWRENCE NOYES

our own best natural resource—our bodies. It is difficult to continue giving to others unless your own physical needs are met and your heart is nourished.

If you are spending a good portion of your time nurturing others through physical contact and touch, make sure you are receiving nurturing touch as well. Find a good massage professional and get sessions as often as you can afford to. Exchange sessions with another practitioner. Trade back rubs or foot massages with another caregiver or volunteer. Sign up with your spouse or a good friend for a relaxation class that includes learning some simple massage techniques so that when the class is over you can continue your "practice" on each other. I have learned the hard way that waiting until one is already on "overload" or in physical pain to pay attention to one's own body is dangerous. When we do not listen to and pay attention to our bodies regularly, we may suddenly find ourselves in a serious health crisis.

SIGNS OF "BURNOUT"

Unrelieved, cumulative stress eventually leads to what has become known in the healthcare community as "burnout," an imbalance in the giving/receiving or working/resting realm of life. Depletion without regeneration leads to burnout. Some ways to avoid the stress that can create such an imbalance include

- recognizing your own limits
- taking good care of your body
- finding ways to feed and nourish your spirit
- learning to identify signs of stress before you get overwhelmed
- periodically looking at your life goals and how what you are doing reflects those goals
- doing things that contribute to those goals
- building a support system
- using relaxation and stress reduction techniques

In my view, it is essential to take the time, on a regular basis, to contemplate what you need in order to maintain a balance in your life. Then, as an ongoing project, work toward creating health and harmony. Try to eat well, get regular exercise, develop a philosophy of living (and dying) that sustains you, and find a productive way of processing your thoughts and feelings as they arise in regard to your work or caregiving responsibilities.

RESOURCES FOR CAREGIVERS

American Association of Retired Persons
    601 E St., N.W.
    Washington, D.C. 20049
    88-424-3410
    www.aarp.org/healthguide

ElderCare Online
    www.ed-online.net
    Chats, resource guides, newsletter, articles

Family Caregiver Alliance
    www.caregiver.org
    Resources on memory loss and brain injury

National Alliance for Caregiving
    4720 Montgomery Lane, Ste. 642, Dept. P
    Bethesda, MD 20814
    www.caregiving.org

National Association for Home Care
    www.nahc.org

Visiting Nurses Association of America
    888-866-8773
    11 Beacon St., Ste. 910, Dept. H
    Boston, MA 02108
    www.vnaa.org

Well Spouse Foundation
    www.wellspouse.org
    Support groups, chats

PROCESSING GRIEF AND INTEGRATING LOSS

If you choose to work with the frail elderly and seriously ill you will be confronted with dying and with death on a regular basis. Dealing with some of your own feelings and issues about aging, illness, death and dying becomes essential. It is another way of taking care of yourself so that you can continue to care for others.

As you relate to those in later life stages, the reality of your experience will afford you a natural avenue to continue your own inner process in regard to these issues. Being confronted with that which is unfamiliar, uncomfortable, threatening and even frightening offers tremendous opportunity for personal and spiritual growth.

Anytime you open your heart to another and let that individual have personal meaning to you, you are also opening yourself to the pain of loss. A unique intimacy can develop fairly quickly between two people in the context of touch sessions. When you have been relating

I used to go to a lot of memorial services. I don't go to as many anymore. I process my grief in my own way. I have friends and family members who also work with the dying and talking with them helps a lot... I consider my patients who have died my guardian angels so I have an abundance of angels.

DOROTHY CHAKNOVA,
C.M.T., HOSPICE HOME HEALTH AIDE

I usually take a little time off after a death. I go to the ocean or the woods, somewhere serene and peaceful and I write a letter to the person who has died.

DEANNA MATTHEWS,
C.M.T., HOSPICE

to another through something as intimate as conscious touch and then the physical form, the vehicle for your contact, is no longer available, feeling bereft is almost inevitable. When the person you have been working with, even for a short period of time, dies, you will be confronted with your own feelings of loss and grief. In addition to your sadness about the end of a particular form of relationship and the knowledge that you will not see that person again, you may feel suddenly "cut off," superfluous or unneeded. The periods of time you spent with that individual each day or week are suddenly empty. The flow of your caring energy toward that person is disrupted. It becomes necessary for you to go through a letting-go process in relation to the person who has died and possibly to other people involved with that person, and to find new ways to channel your energy.

You may or may not be invited to attend a memorial service, or asked to share in the grieving process with the family and close friends of the deceased. If you are working simultaneously with a number of people in later life stages, you will probably not have the time to attend the funeral or memorial service of each one who dies. If you are part of a volunteer organization or caregiving team, you may have the support of group meetings in which you can share your feelings with others who have experienced similar kinds of losses. If such opportunities are not available to you, try to find a supportive friend or loved one who is good at listening without interrupting, evaluating or analyzing what you are saying so that you can express your thoughts and feelings.

If there is something you want to say to the person who has died, you can send those thoughts out mentally. You can sit down and write a letter to that person or compose a dialogue until you feel the conversation you want to have is finished. Though such exercises may seem a bit strange at first, I have found in my own grief work that these and similar techniques can be very helpful.

One "completion" exercise I have found useful is drawn from a Gestalt Therapy technique in which you sit down opposite another human being who, for the sake of the exercise, will represent someone who cannot be physically present to whom you have something to say. You look at the person who has agreed to do this exercise with you as if he or she were the person you want to talk to, and you say everything you wish to say to that individual. Stay with it until you feel "complete" with that person. It may be helpful in getting started to follow a list of beginnings such as

> *I feel angry that...*
> *I am sad because...*
> *I want to tell you that...*
> *Something I never told you is that...*
> *I am glad that...*
> *I am sorry that...*
> *I wish we...*
> *I want to...*
> *I forgive you for...*
> *I forgive myself for...*

The "I" statements will help you talk about yourself and what is true for you rather than making evaluative statements about the other person. If you cannot find someone to sit in the chair, you can put a photograph of the person you want to talk to in the chair or simply visualize in your mind's eye that person in physical form sitting in the chair opposite you as you speak. You may need or want to do the exercise once a day or once a week with the same person in mind, until you feel you have really said everything you want to say to that particular individual.

This kind of exercise supports you in saying goodbye to a friend or loved one who may have died unexpectedly or before you were able to complete some communication. It can also be used to get across something to someone who has moved out of your life or with whom you feel unable to communicate in person. Such an exercise is helpful in integrating change or loss of any kind so that you are freed to move on.

Sometimes writing a poem or composing a song which expresses something about a person who has died, about your interaction with that individual or about your own feelings, can be helpful in a grieving process. You might also choose an art form such as painting, drawing, sculpting or creating a collage to help you access, visualize and express your emotions. These expressions can be kept private or you might decide to share them with family or friends of the deceased, or with other members of the helping community.

There came a time when the deaths of those I was giving touch sessions to were coming much too frequently for me to write something about each person or attend every memorial service. Eventually, I developed the habit of simply sitting in a quiet place, selecting a candle, lighting it and putting my attention on the person who had died.

This ritual can take five minutes or as long as you wish it to. Using the candle as a point of focus, bring the person who has died into your conscious awareness. Think about what you may have learned from your relationship with that individual. Reflect on how you may have grown as a result of your relationship with him or her. Experience your gratitude for those gifts. If you feel the need to say anything else to that person, go ahead and do that, either silently or out loud. You can continue your contemplation until the candle burns itself out or you can leave the candle burning (in a safe container and place) as a way of honoring that person.

Sometimes I plant a new bush in my rose garden in honor of the life of a loved one. Sometimes I do something special for someone else in honor of the person who has left his or her physical body. I don't make a big deal out of it and I usually don't tell anyone else. In my heart I simply dedicate whatever good deed I'm doing to the memory of the particular person I'm think of.

There is no formula, time limit or standard for measuring grief or for adjusting to loss. There is no specific point in time where you stop being sad, where everything is "back to normal" and okay again. Each one of us must forge his or her own path through trauma, change and grief. There is no right or wrong way and the process will take as long as it takes. Our reactions will be slightly different with each loss.

Toward the end of the first day of a workshop I was giving, one of the participants asked to speak with me privately. She began to cry as she told me about the death of her mother and how sad she still felt about this loss. It soon became evident that she was getting feedback from well meaning friends and family, and perhaps internally as well, that enough time had passed since her loss so that she should now be "getting on with her life." She was still 'crying buckets' as she put it, but felt she had to hide this fact from friends and other loved ones who kept congratulating her for getting 'better' and "back to normal." This person had enjoyed a very good and close relationship with her mother and was not grieving for things left unsaid—she simply missed her mother's presence in her life... I did not continue to question this woman. Instead, I simply held her, and accepted her tears.

AUTHOR

The death of a particular friend, family member, patient or client may bring back to you a loss from earlier in your life which you have not yet completely processed. You then have an opportunity for deeper healing and integration. If you are giving touch sessions to someone who reminds you of one of your parents or another loved one who has died, or to a person who is suffering from the same disease as someone you have known and loved, you will probably be more emotionally reactive to that person's illness and eventual death. You will feel the loss more or less intensely depending on how attached you have become to that individual. You may be able to process your feelings fairly quickly or you may integrate the loss slowly over time.

Know that coping with loss, of any kind, takes emotional, mental and psychic energy. When you are actively adjusting to and processing a significant loss, or multiple losses in your life, you may be tired much of the time. Emotional jolts and feelings of deep sadness or anger can arise when you least expect them. You may notice yourself experiencing fear about your own death or the death of loved ones.

There are many creative rituals and exercises for moving through a grief process or for honoring the life of someone who has died. The crucial thing, for your continued mental and emotional health, is to acknowledge the loss you feel and do whatever feels right or appropriate to you to mark the transition that has occurred. Ask for help if necessary and take whatever time you need, use whatever tools you have at your disposal, to assist you in your grieving process. Denial of the emotions connected with grief can lead to dis-ease and to all kind of other physical, mental and emotional problems.

Some years ago I was working with two different women who were suffering from the same type of cancer. Both these women were close to my own age and both had teenage children. The two women were quite different in personality and temperament, and I liked them both. I had been seeing each of these women for only a few weeks when one of them died. The next day, I made a previously unscheduled visit to see the other woman and her husband, because I sensed that she, too, might die soon. As I was driving home that day, I took several wrong turns, ended up on a dead-end street and nearly ran head-on into a large truck! When I got home I switched on the television and began eating nonstop. Later that evening, I was extremely irritable with my husband and daughter. I developed a raging headache, and I could not figure out why I was so tired! I finally recognized that I was doing everything I could to avoid experiencing my grief and my anger at the unfairness of this disabling disease taking women in the prime of life away from their families! I felt such sadness for the daughter of the woman who had died the day before, for her scientist husband, her grieving parents, and her younger sister, all of whom had been helpless against the cancer that so quickly overwhelmed their gentle loved one. I felt the pain of the woman about to die, confronting her death so directly, the woman I had touched and laughed and cried with earlier that day. This woman was six years younger than I, and I had a four-year old child! Those facts scared me. I felt threatened and vulnerable! As soon as I allowed all these thoughts and feelings to surface, allowed myself to release my anger and my tears, opened my heart to my fear and my vulnerability, my headache and fatigue disappeared!

You will find it difficult to be with another's discomfort, whether it be physical pain or mental agony, if you have not allowed yourself to open to the possibility of that same situation occurring in your own life. If you are able to face and accept your own fears and anxieties about aging, illness, death and dying, you will be able to support someone else in facing and accepting his or her fears and feelings of anguish and despair as they arise.

To the extent that you are able to accept your grief, and to bring it into conscious thought and expression, it will dissolve. This is seldom done in one cathartic moment. It happens incrementally in steps and spurts and in its own time. Step by step, whatever you have learned from your experience, whatever you have gained from your interaction with a particular individual can be integrated into your life. Your relationship with that person will then continue to contribute to and enrich your work with others.

Appendix I

Questions and Answers Regarding Touch Sessions

---

1. **Where should I do the touch session?**

   You could do the session anywhere the recipient is comfortable or wherever you find him or her if it seems appropriate. If you are receiving payment for a touch session given in a care facility, federal regulations require that service be provided in the resident's room.

2. **What if the person I am offering the touch session to:**

   a) doesn't want to be touched?

   Never force the physical contact. Remember that you touch a person with the quality of your attention and your presence. Visit, listen, build rapport. Offer some form of touch again in a few minutes and remain open to the individual.

   b) gets up and walks away in the middle of the session?

   Follow the person, holding his or her arm or hand if possible. If the person cannot be persuaded to stop or to sit down, you can give a gentle back rub as you walk. If the person is trying to get away from you, consider this a negative indicator and try making contact again later or the next time you visit.

   c) falls asleep during the session?

   You can usually consider this a positive indicator. Stay with the person, keep your attention on him or her and continue gentle, attentive touch until you feel "complete" or until the agreed upon time for your session is over.

   d) becomes flirtatious during the session?

   Handle this with understanding and humor whenever possible. Make sure your touch is focused and your own intentions are clear.

e) exhibits sexual behavior during the session?

Avoid becoming critical or judgmental of the behavior. Shift the person's focus of attention if possible. Try moving behind the chair and using touch techniques on the shoulders and upper back where you can apply a bit more pressure on larger muscles.

If the behavior continues, let the person know that he or she may need some privacy now and that you will come back later.

f) starts crying during the session?

Accept this as just what is happening. Acknowledge the communication simply without trying to stop the expression or analyzing it too much. This kind of emotional release is common during touch sessions with those in fragile physical and mental states. It is usually a positive indicator. Occasionally it is an involuntary response.

g) becomes agitated during the session?

Keep your attention on the individual. Let your touch be simple and steady. Agitation may indicate that the touch is confusing or overwhelming, or the person is trying to communicate something.

h) tries to hit me during the session?

If possible, move with the flow of the energy rather than resisting or using an opposing force to try to stop the motion until the energy dissipates or you can redirect the movement.

i) becomes verbally or physically abusive during the session?

If you can, ignore talk that simply makes you uncomfortable. Do not let yourself be abused. Leave the room if you need to. Call for help if you need it.

j) won't let go of my hand when I try to end the session?

Acknowledge the communication in some way such as saying, "I'm glad you enjoyed our time together," "I'm sorry I have to go now," or "It's hard to say good-bye sometimes."

Shift the focus of attention to a new object. Give the person something to hold on to such as a pillow or stuffed animal or squeeze ball. Try stroking the top of the hand that is gripping yours. Try timing your session so that some other pleasurable activity coincides with the end of the session.

Appendix II

Dyad Communication Technique

There are advantages to doing a dyad exercise with a facilitator, especially in the beginning. However, a form of the exercise can be done with any other person who is willing to participate with you in the Dyad, following the guidelines outlined below.

BEFORE DOING THE DYAD:

1. Find a time and space where you will be distracted as little as possible

2. Make a mutual decision on what instruction or set of instructions to use.

3. Decide on a length of time for the exercise. (Thirty to forty minutes is good length. In the beginning you can try shorter periods of ten to twenty minutes.)

4. Sit on chairs or on the floor so that you and your partner are on the same level, a comfortable distance apart.

5. Decide on a specific instruction and stick with that wording for the entire exercise.

6. Set a timer or alarm to signal when the time period is over.

RUNNING THE DYAD:

1. Decide who will give the instruction first and who will receive the instruction first, and then begin.

2. As a listening partner: Put your attention on your partner before giving the instruction. Give your full and undivided attention to the person communicating. Remain open to your partner and in contact with him or her. Listen without interrupting or commenting on anything your partner says. Speak only to say "clarify" if you do not hear or understand something that is said. When you have received and understood your partner's communication say "thank you" and give the next instruction to your partner (or reverse roles if you are using only one instruction).

3. As a communicating partner: Take time to receive the instruction (let it sink into your consciousness). Contemplate (ponder, consider) the instruction given. Tell your partner what occurred when you contemplated the instruction – communicate any thoughts, bodily sensations or feelings, etc. that came up

as a result of contemplating the instruction and leave out any other thoughts that were unrelated to that. Get across one complete thought at a time each time it is your turn to communicate (rather than all your thoughts on the subject all at once).

- Be as concise as you can.
- Use words and anything else you need to get the communication across.
- When you have complied with the instruction given, wait for an acknowledgment from your partner, then receive the next instruction, or reverse roles.
- After your partner says "thank you," wait for the second part of the instruction or reverse roles and give your partner the same instruction you received.

Some Sample Instructions:

Two-part instructions:

A. Tell me something you like about your job.

B. Tell me something that is difficult for you about your job.

A. Tell me a concern you have about aging.

B. Tell me a fear you have about dying.

Single Instructions:

Tell me what death means to you.

Tell me what you fear most about dying.

Tell me how (someone's) death affected you.

Note: Even though each partner will have the opportunity to communicate about a number of concerns or fears over the course of the exercise, repeat the instruction, "Tell me a concern… " or "Tell me a fear… " each time to make it fresh and precise.

When you have completed the Dyad exercise, avoid analyzing, commenting on, or going into dialogue with your partner or others about anything that was said during the exercise.

Appendix III

10 Warning Signs of Alzheimer's disease

The Alzheimer's Association has developed a list of warning signs that include common symptoms of Alzheimer disease (some also apply to other types of dementia). If someone you know has several of these symptoms, he or she should see a physician for a complete examination.

1. Memory loss that affects job skills. It's normal to occasionally forget an assignment, deadline or colleague's name, but frequent forgetfulness or unexplainable confusion at home or in the workplace may signal that something's wrong.

2. Difficulty performing familiar tasks. Busy people get distracted from time to time. For example, you might leave something on the stove too long or not remember to serve part of a meal. People with Alzheimer's might prepare a meal and not only forget to serve it but also forget they made it.

3. Problems with language. Everyone has trouble finding the right word sometimes, but a person with Alzheimer's disease may forget simple words or substitute inappropriate words, making his or her sentences difficult to understand.

4. Disorientation to time and place. It's normal to momentarily forget the day of the week or what you need from the store. But people with Alzheimer's disease can become lost on their own street, not knowing where they are, how they got there, or how to get back home.

5. Poor or decreased judgment. Choosing not to bring a sweater or coat along on a chilly night is a common mistake. A person with Alzheimer's, however, may dress inappropriately in more noticeable ways, wearing a bathrobe to the store or several blouses on a hot day.

6. Problems with abstract thinking. Balancing a checkbook can be challenging for many people, but for someone with Alzheimer's, recognizing numbers or performing basic calculation may be impossible.

7. Misplacing things. Everyone temporarily misplaces a wallet or keys from time to time. A person with Alzheimer's disease may put these and other items in inappropriate places — such as an iron in the freezer or a wristwatch in the sugar bowl and then not recall how they got there.

8. Changes in mood or behavior. Everyone experiences a broad range of emotions — it's part of being human. People with Alzheimer's tend to exhibit more rapid mood swings for no apparent reason.

9. Changes in personality. People's personalities may change somewhat as they age. But a person with Alzheimer's can change dramatically, either suddenly or over a period of time. Someone who is generally easygoing may become angry, suspicious, or fearful.

10. Loss of initiative. It's normal to tire of housework, business activities, or social obligations, but most people retain or eventually regain their interest. The person with Alzheimer's disease may remain uninterested and uninvolved in many or all of his usual pursuits.

Source: Alzheimer's Disease and Related Disorders Association, Inc. 919 North Michigan Avenue, Suite 1100 Chicago, Illinois 60611-1676 (800)-272-3900 www.alz.org

Annotated Bibliography

Books for Adults

This particular listing contains books that have contributed to my personal and professional growth, that I have found useful, over the last decade, in writing about, practicing and teaching COMPASSIONATE TOUCH® and that I recommend to students, clients or caregivers.

Published books dealing specifically with the efficacy of touch in caring for the elderly and the ill are few and far between. This particular form of therapeutic contact is often ignored or given short shrift in healthcare books and in books about caregiving and about death and dying. Happily, articles on this subject are appearing much more frequently than they were when I wrote my first book in 1993 and groundbreaking books such as *Medicine Hands* by Gayle MacDonald have been published. This bibliography is by no means exhaustive, and there are certainly other excellent books available on some of the subjects mentioned.

TOUCH AND MASSAGE

Care Through Touch: Massage as the Art of Anointing by Mary Ann Finch (New York: Continuum Publishing, 1999).

> Offered by its author as "a gift to the marginalized men, women and children who are the forgotten members of society: the homeless, the frail and isolated elderly, the poor, the dying, the mentally ill, the addict," this book speaks to the heart of healing. A valuable resource offering support, guidance and inspiration to massage students, professional bodyworkers, volunteers and anyone interested in integrating touch into his or her caregiving role.

Healing Massage Techniques: Holistic, Classic and Emerging Methods by Frances M. Tappan (New York: Appleton and Lange, 1988).

> For those who want to learn more about the history and purposes of massage, this book describes an array of massage techniques along with principles, procedures and applications. A section on the use of massage for various healing purposes has a short segment on the use of massage in nursing.

Healing Touch: A Complete Guide to the Use of Touch Therapies that Promote Well Being by Marcus and Maria Webb (New York: Sterling Publishing Company, 1999).

> This well-organized, color illustrated book offers an overview of various hands-on treatments available today including their history, philosophy and application. Includes advice for treating children.

Healing Touch: The Church's Forgotten Language by Zach Thomas (Westminster/John Knox Press, 1994).

> Thomas writes from his unique perspective as a Presbyterian minister, a former hospital chaplain and a professional bodyworker, sharing insights based on extensive study and experience. His book advocates reclaiming the ancient practice of healing touch and presents biblical principles as a model for touch in pastoral care. The author elucidates the power of healing touch which he defines as "an important way of sharing compassion" in in three main areas—caring relationships, professional settings and worship.

The Massage Book by George Downing, illustrated by Anne Ken Rush (New York: Random House, 1972).

> One of the first books, and still one of the best, published on the art and practice of basic therapeutic massage. Though this book does not deal specifically with the subject of massaging the elderly or the ill, it remains an excellent introduction to massage as a tool for stress reduction and relaxation.

Massage Therapy Guidelines for Hospital and Home Care, 4th ed. by Tedi Dunn and Marian Williams (available through Information for People, Olympia, WA, 1-800-754-9790)

> A welcome guidebook for massage therapists wishing to find their place in hospitals and other health-care environments and for the administrators and organizations who wish to support them. Includes guidelines for hospital-based massage, models for implementing massage programs in medical settings and copies of articles by pioneers in the field.

Medicine Hands: Massage Therapy for People with Cancer by Gayle MacDonald (Findhorn, Scotland: Findhorn Press, 1999).

> Well-researched, well-written and thorough, this unique and beautifully formatted book is chock-full of intelligent advice, practical wisdom and inspirational stories. There is also invaluable information in the Appendixes such as a Glossary of Bodywork Modalities, lists of organizations and publications and so on. A much needed and much welcomed resource for massage professionals and for all caregivers!

The Power of Touch by Phyllis K. Davis (Carson, California: Hay House, 1991).

> Written by a professional counselor and communications consultant, this book discusses different kinds of touch, attitudes toward touch in American society and how touch makes a difference in people's lives. The book includes activities and exercises for self-reflection.

The Therapeutic Touch: How to Use Your Hands to Help or to Heal by Dolores Krieger, Ph.D., R.N. (New York: Prentice-Hall, 1979).

> This book, a classic in the field, has helped countless numbers of people since its inception. Ms. Krieger believes that we all have the potential of directing human energy through our hands to help and heal ourselves and others. Her book contains a number of "self-knowledge tests" which are useful as centering practices and in learning how to detect and direct energy. Also included are numerous case histories and examples of the use of Therapeutic Touch as defined by the author.

Touching: The Human Significance of the Skin by Ashley Montagu (New York: Harper and Row, 1971, 1978, 1986).

> In this remarkable book, a renowned anthropologist examines the significance of touch and its relationship to well-being and documents the importance of tactile interaction on human development. The author discusses the relationship of the skin and touching to physical and mental health and includes a thought-provoking chapter on the importance of touch for older people.

Where Healing Waters Meet: Touching Mind and Emotion through the Body by Clyde W. Ford (New York: Station Hill Press, 1989).

> An important book for anyone practicing a touch-based therapy. Drawing from personal and profession therapeutic experience, Ford, a chiropractor, explores and elucidates the powerful connection between the body and the mind and how that configuration can support healing.

CAREGIVING

Arthritis Relief at Your Fingertips by Michael Reed Gach (New York: Warner Books, 1989).

> This book is a gold mine for the 35 million Americans suffering from arthritis and rheumatism and for anyone who works with the elderly. The self-help techniques outlined in this book provide relief to the victims of these crippling diseases. The clear photos and line drawings that accompany the text make it easy to learn and use the techniques which can be taught or incorporated into massage or touch sessions. Cassette tapes with guidance for daily practice are also available.

Caring For An Elderly Relative: A Guide to Home Care by M. Keith Thompson, M.D. (New York: Prentice-Hall, 1986).

> This practical and informative book contains many helpful hints about caring for and relating to older people. It details some of the specific issues and challenges inherent in aging on both the physical and mental levels.

Caring For Your Aging Parents by Barbara Deane (NavPress, 1989).

> A chapter in this book "Coping with the Heath Problems of the Aging" is particularly helpful to those working with the elderly and/or the ill in that it describes diseases which are common in later life stages, giving symptoms, common treatments and possible side effects of some of those treatments.

ALZHEIMER'S DISEASE

The Alzheimer's Sourcebook for Care-givers: A Practical Guide for Getting Through the Day by Frena Gray Davidson (Los Angeles: Lowell House, 1993).

> A client of mine told me that this book helped her immensely in caring for her mother at home in the last two years of her life and recommended it highly. This book not only helps the reader understand what is happening to the person experiencing Alzheimer's disease but gives practical advice and support in finding solutions to daily problems.

Discovering Adventure in Special Care by Rosemary Dunne (Vancouver, B.C.: G.F. Murray, 1998).

> Written by a recreational therapist, this thought-provoking and insightful book reminds the reader to see the individual inside the dementia and offers creative suggestions for affirming and celebrating each person's uniqueness while making sure he or she is safe and cared for. The book is uplifting and inspiring. Following the author's approach will surely enrich the lives of caregivers as well as those who are receiving care.

Speaking Our Minds: Personal Reflections from Individuals with Alzheimer's by Lisa Snyder (New York: W. H. Freeman, 2000).

> This book offers a unique look at Alzheimer's disease through the eyes of men and women who have the disease. Their reflections, along with the author's analytical narrative provide great insight from a rarely heard perspective, on the experience of living with Alzheimer's for both the person with the disease and the family caregivers. This compelling book is written sensitively and positively and is an invaluable resource for family caregivers and anyone wishing to better understand some of the challenges inherent in living with Alzheimer's or taking care of someone with Alzheimer's.

Therapeutic Caregiving: A Practical Guide for Caregivers of Persons with Alzheimer's and Other Dementia Causing Diseases by Barbara J. Bridges, R.N. (Millcreek, Washington: BJB Publishing, 1995).

> A superb, experienced-based book, by a woman who spent thirteen years caring for two parents and a best friend living with dementia. This well-written and well-organized book combines professional expertise with practical advice. It is an excellent resource for anyone facing the formidable task of caring for someone with Alzheimer's or other dementia related conditions.

The 36-Hour Day: A Family Guide to Caring for Persons with Alzheimer's Disease, Related Dementing Illnesses, and Memory Loss in Later Life by Nancy L. Mace and Peter Rabins (Baltimore: John Hopkins Univ. Press, rev. ed. 1991).

> One of the first and best comprehensive guidebooks written, this book is an excellent blueprint for those who find themselves relating in any way to someone with progressive dementia. It contains a wealth of material and gives sound and sage advice on almost every aspect of care. An informative, thorough, practical and invaluable resource.

Alzheimer's Disease: A Practical Guide for Families and Other Caregivers by Judah Ronch (New York: Continuum, 1991).

> A well-written and informative book which gives wise and practical advice and supports caregivers in accepting and respecting the person who is suffering from Alzheimer's disease while facing the challenge of living with or caring for such a person.

CANCER

Making Friends with Cancer by Dawn Nelson (Findhorn, Scotland: Findhorn Press, 2000).

> Though I cannot really be objective in describing this particular book, I would say it is useful for anyone who has cancer, knows someone who has cancer, or is concerned about being diagnosed with cancer or any other life-threatening disease. It shares one person's experience of diagnosis and treatment, encourages conscious decision-making and presents positive and life-affirming ways of dealing with the reality of cancer.

Making the Chemotherapy Decision by David Drum (Los Angeles: Lowell House, 1996).

> This book contains a great deal of good advice and pragmatic suggestions about tolerating chemotherapy treatment and coping with its side effects. Useful for patients, family members and caregivers alike, it will give those working with cancer patients a better understanding of what is involved in the decision making process as well as in undergoing chemotherapy treatment.

When a Parent Has Cancer: A Guide to Caring for Your Children by Wendy Schlessel Harpham (New York: HarperCollins, 1997).

> The author, mother of three, a physician and a cancer survivor, writes with authority, honesty and clarity that can come only from direct experience. Full of useful and pragmatic advice for parents with children of all ages, the book is also encouraging and comforting. Included, as an insert, is an excellent little book, *Becky and the Worry Cup* for children to read alone or together with a parent.

When Life Becomes Precious: A Guide for Loved Ones and Friends of Cancer Patients by Elise NeeDell Babcock (New York: Bantam Books, 1997).

> An excellent resource with hundreds of practical and applicable tips for friends, family members and caregivers of those experiencing cancer or any other serious illness. One of the best chapters includes a list "52 Gifts You Can Give" to offer support to those living with cancer.

When Someone You Love Has Cancer: What You Must Know, What You Can Do, What You Should Expect by Suzanne LeVert (New York: Dell Publishing, 1995).

> Informative, concise, straightforward and practical book that I often recommend to people who wonder what to do or how they can help, or to those who simply feel lost when a family member or a friend receives a cancer diagnosis.

When Your Friend Gets Cancer: How You Can Help, by Amy Harwell with Kristine Tomasik (Wheaton, Illinois: Harold Shaw Publishers, 1987).

> An easy-to-read and practical book that offers sensible and compassionate guidance on how to be a friend and what you can do when someone you love has cancer.

APPROACHING DEATH

AIDS The Ultimate Challenge by Elisabeth Kubler-Ross (New York: MacMillan, 1987).

> This unique book challenges, inspires and educates the reader in regard to every aspect of what may be the world's most serious health crisis—the AIDS epidemic. Irene Smith, who Kubler-Ross calls her "pride and joy" and who began massaging people with AIDS in 1982 when many people were afraid to touch them, writes in a very honest and moving way in one section in this book about the emotional and spiritual impact of her early years in caring for those dying of AIDS.

Close to the Bone: Life Threatening Illness and the Search for Meaning by Jean Shinoda Bolen (New York: Touchstone, 1998).

> Dr. Bolen's rich understanding of the human condition, in both archetypal and individual form, inhabits all her books. In this book she details the value of illness, loss and death viewed as a soul journey, or spiritual initiation, drawing from the experiences of clients and friends as well as from her own life.

Healing into Life and Death by Stephen Levine (New York: Anchor Press/Doubleday, 1987).

> Like all Stephen's books, this one is thought provoking and investigative into the nature of what true healing is. Techniques are offered for working with pain and grief and for developing merciful awareness in regard to ourselves and those with whom we come in contact. A compassionate guide.

Home Care for the Dying by Deborah Whiting Little (New York: Doubleday, 1985).

> Certain sections of this book give practical guidance and useful information for anyone who might be involved in serving or helping care for someone who is ill and/or elderly in a home setting. This book also addresses the issue of stress faced by family members caring for a loved one who is facing death.

The Hospice Handbook A New Way To Care For The Dying, ed. by Michael Hamilton and Helen Reid (William B. Eerdmans Publishing, 1980).

> A good resource book for anyone interested in working with hospice patients or with the dying in general. Gives a history of the hospice concept and goals. The personal essays in Part I are particularly useful in providing insight into the needs of the seriously ill. Part III explains the elements of organization and outlines some of the differences between hospice, hospital and nursing home care.

Meetings at the Edge: Dialogues with the Grieving and the Dying, the Healing and the Healed by Stephen Levine (New York: Anchor Press/Doubleday 1984).

> For a period of about three years, the author and his wife, Ondrea, offered a free consultation phone for the "terminally ill and those working closely with a death." This book is a sharing of a number of those conversations. The dialogues are intimate, moving and instructive.

Tuesdays with Morrie: An Old Man, a Young Man, and Life's Greatest Lessons by Mitch Albom (New York: Doubleday, 1997).

> In this wise and wonderful book, the author shares the courage, insight and wisdom of Morrie Schwartz, his favorite college professor, who, years later, is facing death from ALS. Albom passes on the gift of his last tutorial from this great teacher in this unique and moving book, which has much to teach us all.

To Live Until We Say Good-Bye, text by Elisabeth Kubler-Ross, photographs by Mal Warshaw (New York: Prentice-Hall, 1978).

> A profoundly moving and compassionate work which contains thought-provoking text along with heart-opening visual images of individuals of different ages who, along with their loved ones, volunteers and friends, share their process in facing life-threatening illness and death. This book is intimate, positive and powerfully eloquent.

Who Dies? An Investigation of Conscious Living and Conscious Dying by Stephen Levine (New York: Anchor Press/Doubleday, 1982).

> This book is just what the title says it is. Read with an open mind and heart, it might change one's perspective about living and about dying significantly. Essential, though not "easy," reading for any serious student of life/death.

GRIEF AND BEREAVEMENT

I Never Know What To Say: How to Help Your Family and Friends Cope with Tragedy by Nina Herrmann Donnelley (New York: Ballentine Books, 1987).

> A book that is helpful in its personal insights about facing death, the various aspects of mourning a loss and what to say to others who are grieving. It contains a short section on the importance of touching those who are ill or dying.

The Courage To Grieve: Creative Living, Recovery, & Growth Through Grief by Judy Tatelbaum (New York: Harper and Row, 1980).

> An excellent and truly useful book, well written with compassion and sensitivity, on all aspects of grief and grief resolution. A valuable aid to anyone who works with the aged, the seriously ill and the grieving.

Good Grief Rituals: Tools for Healing by Elaine Childs-Gowell (New York: Station Hill Press, 1992).

> This is a gentle little book that contains simple exercises that can support one in dealing with loss of any kind. It presents a treasure box of tools for help in the integration and healing process.

You Don't Have to Suffer: A Handbook for Moving Beyond Life's Crises by Judy Tatelbaum (New York: Harper and Row, 1989). Currently out of print.

> The author offers a discerning analysis on suffering and how it can be overcome and useful support for moving out of self-destructive thoughts and emotions.

When Your Friend is Grieving: Building a Bridge of Love by Paula D'Arcy (Wheaton, Illinois: Harold Shaw Publishers, 1990).

> An excellent resource for supporting anyone who is in a grief process. Written by a woman following the sudden death of her husband and child, this book gives specific and practical suggestions for what to say, what not to say and what one can do for a friend who is grieving.

SELF-CARE/INSPIRATION

Acupressure's Potent Points: A Guide to Self-Care for Common Ailments by Michael Reed Gach (New York: Bantam, 1990)

> This book makes the ancient healing art of finger pressure accessible in the modern world. The author reveals simple, learnable techniques which enable the reader to relieve more than forty common ailments and symptoms using the power and sensitivity of his or her own hands. Photographs of real people practicing the techniques outlined in the text, as well as easy-to-read line drawings enhance this book.

Kitchen Table Wisdom: Stories That Heal by Rachel Naomi Remen, M.D. (New York: Riverhead Books, 1996).

> From her personal experience as a physician, a pioneer in the mind/body health field and a long-term survivor of chronic illness, the author shares stores about living and dying, loving and laughing, listening and learning, helping and healing. The book is authentic, personal, powerful and inspirational, offering food for the heart and for the soul.

Natural Health, Natural Medicine: A Comprehensive Manual for Wellness and Self-Care by Andrew Weil, M.D. (Boston: Houghton Mifflin, 1990).

> Working within the medical profession and advocating natural medicine and self-care as a legitimate alternative to conventional medical treatment, Dr. Weil has compiled a great deal of information into a practical, clear, readable and highly useful health guide. An invaluable resource for health maintenance, the book outlines specific preventive measures to take in order to avoid debilitating diseases and protect the immune system.

SERVICE AND HEALING

Guided Meditations, Explorations and Healings by Stephen Levine (New York: Anchor Books/Doubleday, 1991).

> Guided meditations, mindfulness practices and processes for self awareness and to use for exploration and relaxation in working with others. Any of the meditations can be adapted to your own style and then read aloud or recorded on tape for those you work with to listen to.

Healers On Healing, ed. by Richard Carlson and Benjamin Shield (New York: Jeremy P. Tarcher, 1989).

> This important work is an anthology of essays written by nearly forty different well-known, non-traditional physicians and healers who explore the nature of healing from various viewpoints. Some of the topics addressed include love as a healing force, the effects of healing relationships, the power of the healer within, healing and death, and how healing takes place.

The Helper's Journey by Dale G. Larson (Champaign, Illinois: Research Press, 1993).

> Drawing from the worlds of hospice, nursing, education and counseling, this book explores theoretical as well as the practical aspects of caregiving. The author offers specific techniques and strategies to help caregivers deal with stress, avoid burnout and cope with other challenges.

How Can I Help? Stories and Reflections on Service by Ram Dass and Paul Gorman (New York: Alfred A. Knopf, 1986).

> This is a book I refer to again and again. Thought-provoking, insightful and instructive, it offers practical guidance as well as inspiration, through deeply moving personal stories of caring and compassion. A "must read" for anyone interested in serving others and deepening compassion.

FOR MASSAGE PROFESSIONALS

Business Mastery by Cherie Sohnen-Moe (Tucson, Arizona: Sohnen-Moe Assoc., 1991).

> Created especially for self-employed professionals in the healing arts, this book is a guide for creating a fulfilling, successful business based on "creativity, joy, empowerment, balance and profitability." A valuable resource for anyone who wants to achieve success in a service-oriented business.

Therapeutic Massage in Facility Care: Benefits, Effects and Implementation by Dawn Nelson and Brianna Allen (Tallahassee, Florida: Findhorn Press, 2001; pre-published format available through Information for People at 1-800-754-9790).

> Details the benefits of massage programs for both residents and staff in care facilities and offers valuable guidelines for creating and implementing such programs. Includes sample contracts, authorization, documentation and other forms.

EDUCATIONAL VIDEOS

The Power of Touch in Facility Care – 10 min.

Compassionate Touch: Benefits and Effects in Long Term Care – 23 min.

Compassionate Touch: Benefits and Effects in Alzheimer's Care – 27 min.

The award-winning videos above by AllenTouch Productions are available through Information for People (1-800-754-9790)

The Emotional Impact of Working with the Dying (Irene Smith) available through Health Positive at www.healthpositive.com or phone 1-888-797-5594

Books for Children

About Dying: An Open Family Book for Parents and Children Together by Sara Bonnett Stein (New York: Walker and Company, 1974).

> This book is one of a series designed to help adults help young children, ages 2 to 6, in dealing with challenging life situations. It introduces the subject of death, dying and grieving a loss through simple, honest words and realistic photographs relating to the death of a pet bird and then a grandfather. The accompanying text for adults acts as a springboard for questions that may arise during the reading of the book with a child by giving suggestions for more specific and detailed discussion.

Badger's Parting Gifts by Susan Varley (New York: Mulberry Books, 1984).

> Tired old Badger feels as though his body does not work as well as it used to and that death is most likely nearing. That night he has an unusual dream about running down a Long Tunnel. There is a liberating and joyful feeling attached to this event, which is actually Badger's death. Badger's animal friends gather together and begin to share stories about the special memories they have of Badger. The friends all tell each other of something learned, a "Gift" from Badger they will always have and can pass on. This unique story, for ages 3 to 9, emphasizes the positive aspects and lasting value of a life well lived as well as suggesting an important technique for sharing grief and integrating loss.

Everett Anderson's Goodbye by Lucille Clifton, illus. Ann Grifalconi (New York: Henry Holt 1983).

> Written in verse, this book is about a little boy's struggles through what Elizabeth Kubler-Ross termed the five stages of grief—denial, anger, bargaining, depression, acceptance—after the death of his Daddy. The wonderful pencil drawings are a powerful and integral part of the simple and empathetic poetry, which expresses this small boy's emotions quite powerfully.

The Fall of Freddie the Leaf: A Story of Life for All Ages by Leo Buscaglia (New Jersey: Charles B. Slack, 1982).

> A wonderfully wise book that tells the story of a leaf named Freddie, following the changes which Freddie and his leaf friend and teacher, Daniel, undergo from their "birth" in Spring to their "death" in Winter. Illustrated with beautiful photographs of trees and leaves during the changing seasons of the year. A treasure for any age and any season, and an excellent first book for introducing young children to death as part of the natural flow of life in all forms.

I'll Always Love You by Hans Wilheim (New York: Crown Publications, 1989).

> A wonderful and charming picture book suitable for young children, aged 3 to 8, grieving over the death of a pet or over any death. This book introduces the very important concept of communicating our feelings to those we love while they are alive! It also illustrates the importance of support and of sharing our sadness.

Lifetimes: The Beautiful Way to Explain Death to Children by Bryan Mellonie & Robert Ingpen (New York: Bantam Books, 1983).

> This beautifully written book uses a young child's fascination with birds, fish, insects, plants and people to explain that all living things have lifetimes and that dying is as much a part of living as

being born. The text is simple and sensitive and the illustrations are large and lovely. It emphasizes that lifetimes are different lengths for different kinds of animals and for different people and that what they have is common is a beginning, an ending and the time in between.

Last Week My Brother Anthony Died by Martha Whitmore, Illus. by Randie Julien (Abington Press, 1984).

This is one of the few books I've seen which speaks to the specific situation of the death of a baby as seen through the eyes of a sibling. A little girl named Julie narrates the story, describing her feelings after the death of her four-week-old baby brother.

Losing Someone You Love: When a Brother or Sister Dies. Text and photos by Elizabeth Richter (New York: G. P. Putnam's Sons, 1986).

For older children who have lost a sibling to death, this book could be an invaluable resource. Fifteen individuals between the ages of ten and twenty tell their personal stories. A photograph accompanies each story.

The Mountains of Tibet by Mordicai Gerstein (New York: Harper and Row, 1987).

If you believe in reincarnation as an after death experience, you will find this book a gentle treasure! The back cover says "ages 7 up" but it was one of my youngest daughter's favorite books when she was three. Beautifully written and illustrated and full of possibility.

My Grandma Leonie by Bijou Le Tord (New York: Bradbury Press, 1987).

This sweet and reassuring book for a young child encourages quiet sharing. The simple text is accompanied by delicate watercolor paintings. The child narrates, describing all the things she did with her grandmother and how she felt when her grandmother died. When she missed her grandma, she would "sit in a chair, turn on the radio and think of how much she loved me."

Sadako and the Thousand Paper Cranes by Eleanor Coerr, Paintings by Ronald Himler (New York: A Dell Yearling Book, 1977).

The remarkable and true story of a Japanese girl who died at age twelve, as a result of radiation from the bomb dropped on Hiroshima when she was two years old is told in a straightforward and tender way, without drama or morbidity. The Japanese have a saying that if a sick person folds a thousand paper cranes, the gods will grant her wish and make her well again. With the encouragement of her friends and family, Sadako begins the project. Having folded 644 cranes when she dies, her classmates fold the rest.

The Sky Goes on Forever: a Book about Death for Children written and illustrated by Molly MacGregor (Clearlake, California: Dawn Horse Press, 1989).

A thoughtful and thought-provoking book which gently introduces a spiritual perspective to death. It could be read to younger children, aged four to eight, or by or with older children. The book raises important questions and introduces the concept of continuing to communicate with someone after death and emphasizes the importance of love and forgiveness both before and after someone dies.

The Tenth Good Thing About Barney by Judith Viorst, Illust by Erik Belgvad (New York: MacMillan, 1971).

This book has become a classic in children's literature on this subject. When a little boy's beloved cat, Barney, dies, he consoles himself, as his mother suggests, by trying to think of the ten best things about his cat.

Wilfrid Gordon McDonald Partridge by Mem Fox, illus. by Julie Vevis (Kane/Miller Book Publishers, 1985).

A tender and touching story about a little boy who develops a special friendship with a ninety-six-year-old resident of the nursing home next door to his house. Beautifully and humorously illustrated, this charming book teaches invaluable lessons about caring and sharing, while introducing children to the process of aging and memory loss.

References

1 Dolores Krieger, *The Therapeutic Touch: How to Use Your Hands to Help or to Heal* (Prentice-Hall, 1979), 15.

2 Zach Thomas, *The Healing Touch: The Church's Forgotten Language* (Westminster/John Knox Press, 1994), 107.

3 Janet F. Quinn, *Healers on Healing* (Los Angeles: J.P. Tarcher, 1989), 142

4 Thomas, *The Healing Touch*, 15.

5 Edward A. Charlesworth and Ronald G. Nathan, *Stress Management: A Comprehensive Guide to Wellness* (Ballantine Books, 1991), 10.

6 Ibid.

7 Ashley Montagu, *Touching: The Human Significance of the Skin, 3rd ed.* (Harper and Row, 1986), 398.

8 Donna Swanson quoted in *Images, Women in Transition* (St. Mary's College Press, 1977).

9 Quoted in Jon Kabat-Zinn, *Full Catastrophe Living: Using the Wisdom of Your Body and Mind to Face Stress, Pain, and Illness* (Delta, 1990), 215.

10 Lawrence Noyes, personal conversation, January, 1996.

11 Barry Barankin, personal conversation, July, 1999.

12 Susan Jacobsen, written communication, March, 1996.

13 Ibid.

14 Ibid.

15 Rachel Naomi Remen, *Kitchen Table Wisdom:Stories That Heal* (Riverhead Books, 1994).

16 Ram Dass and Paul Gorman, *How Can I Help? Stories and Reflections on Service* (Alfred A. Knopf, 1986), 18.

17 Ibid., 19.

18 Thomas, *Healing Touch*, 15.

19 Montagu, *Touching*: 399.

20 Ibid., 396.

21 Tiffany Field, Key Note Address at AMTA National Convention, November 1997.

22 Alzheimer's Association pamphlet: "Steps to Getting a Diagnosis," 1997.

23 Ibid., 6.

24 Ibid., 7.

25 Alzheimer's Association pamphlet: "Alzheimer's Disease and Related Disorders: A Description of the Dementias," 1997.

26 Alzheimr's Association Ronald & Nancy Reagan Research Institute pamplet: "A World Without Alzheimer's Disease: A Dream Within Reach."

[27] Alzheimer's Association pamphlet: "You Can Make a Difference," 1995.

[28] Cynthia Belle, 4th National Alzheimer's Disease Education Conference presentation, Chicago, Illinois, July, 1995.

[29] Lisa Snyder, *Speaking Our Minds: Personal Reflections from Individuals with Alzheimer's,* (W.H. Freeman and Co., 2000), 23.

[30] Ibid.

[31] Irene Smith, "Bodywork for People with HIV," *Bodywork and Massage Quarterly* (Spring 1994), 43.

[32] Gayle MacDonald, *Medicine Hands: Massage Therapy for People with Cancer,* (Findhorn Press, 1999), 118.

[33] Remen, *Kitchen Table Wisdom,* 255.

[34] Megan Carnarius, *American Health Magazine* (June, 1996), 29.

[35] Liz Madelin, "An Integrated Care Programme," *The International Journal of Aromatherapy,* vol. 6, no. 4.

[36] Dr. Stephan Betz, personal conversation, May, 2001.

[37] Remen, *Kitchen Table Wisdom,* 132.

Acknowledgments

I have been blessed in the past decade to come into relationship with many people whom I would never have met had I not made a decision to provide touch to the confined elderly and ill. I am grateful beyond measure to the women and men who became my teachers by allowing me to touch their bodies, listen to their stories and share their precious time. This book could not have been written without these unique individuals. Very few of them still inhabit their physical bodies yet they live on in my heart.

I wish also to express my gratitude to the family members and caregivers who have opened their homes and their hearts to me; to the care facility administrators and staff members, healthcare professionals, respite center directors, massage school owners, hospice supervisors and chaplains; and to the workshop sponsors who have supported COMPASSIONATE TOUCH® since its inception in 1991; and to those who continue to participate in COMPASSIONATE TOUCH® workshops.

I am especially grateful to the colleagues, students, friends and caregivers who have taken the time to share their personal experiences about the power of touch with me. The desire to pass along their stories was the original inspiration for this book. The stories that do not appear on these particular pages are no less important than the ones that are included; and they are tucked away in my files and in my heart for future sharing.

I express my continued gratitude to several photographers who generously contributed their time as well as the images they captured on film to help enhance the text of this book as well as my first one.

I thank the other photographers, both professional and amateur, who contributed pictures: Brianna Allen, Hunter Bahnson, Barry Barankin, Bonnie Burt, James Patrick Dawson, Karl Mondon and Brock Palmer.

I have been most fortunate to come into contact with Thierry and Karin Bogliolo of Findhorn Press. They and their staff have supported me with generosity, grace and kindness in our joint creation of two books. Both Thierry Bogliolo and Pam Bochel have been especially patient with me through these birthing processes.

My oldest daughter Brianna, encouraged me to create the COMPASSIONATE TOUCH® Program and has helped support my work with the elderly for over a decade. I continue to be inspired by her compassion, her commitment and her skills as a healthcare professional.

I could not work, write, teach or grow without the support of my family. Their presence and their love nurture, sustain and enrich my life daily.

Index

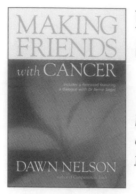

Making Friends with Cancer
by Dawn Nelson

"I received Dawn's manuscript at a time when our own family was facing a life threatening health crisis. What a great gift. This work speaks directly to my feelings and will do so to any who find themselves in the inevitable confrontation with our own mortality. I am grateful for this record and wholeheartedly recommend it to others."
—Helen Palmer, author of The Enneagram

"Making Friends with Cancer is a heartfelt, powerful, poignant and inspiring book. By sharing her own story and determined approach, the author gives cancer patients a positive way of dealing with loss."
—Kirsti A. Dyer, MD, MS, Physician, Internal Medicine

"Making Friends with Cancer is a masterfully woven tapestry of events which allows the reader the opportunity to participate in the author's choice to heal herself, one thought at a time."
—Irene Smith, Founder, Service Through Touch

"Like many folk, I have the underlying thought that if and when I get cancer, my life will be over. Dawn's transformation in befriending cancer and welcoming the gifts it offered her demonstrates the remarkable possibilities open to us all if we too could live in the present and embrace love instead of fear."
—Daniel M. Karan, Ph.D., D.C

Sometimes it becomes imperative for our survival to find new ways to perceive and interpret life's challenges, to let go of old or habitual patterns in order to make informed decisions and conscious commitments in the present. There is no right or wrong answer. Each of us must navigate her or his own way through the formidable waters of something as alarming as a cancer diagnosis, whether that diagnosis is our own or has become the plight of someone we love. We have the power to choose our own response in any situation. The choices we make may not be the popular choices or the most agreed upon choices, but they must be the choices that are authentic for us. They must be the choices that empower rather than subdue us, and they must be choices for which we are willing to take responsibility.

Perhaps we should not be so much concerned with the length of our lives as with its quality. The worst diagnosis of all could be an unlived life. The important query is not how long my lifetime will be in years or what I will die of. The significant questions are:

- Am I still growing? • Am I learning? • Am I loving well? • Am I helping others?
- Am I making healthy, conscious choices? • Am I contributing in some way to making the world a safer, saner place for all of us? • Am I awake? • Am I present?
- Am I saying yes to life now?

This book will speak to any open minded reader who has cancer, fears getting cancer or who loves someone who has cancer. Beyond that, it will speak to anyone who seeks to live in harmony with the way things actually are rather than in habitual resistance to the way things appear to be. You make friends with cancer not by hating it or fighting with it but by acknowledging it as a teacher, accepting what it has to teach you, and continuing on your Journey, one step at a time.

PUBLISHED BY FINDHORN PRESS — BY THE SAME AUTHOR AS FROM THE HEART THROUGH THE HANDS
ISBN 1-899171-38-X

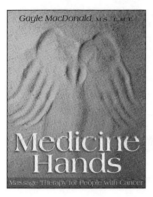

Medicine Hands:
Massage Therapy for People with Cancer
by Gayle MacDonald, M.s., L.M.T.

"...an excellent resource which has long been needed by health professionals. It is full of wise advice for both patients and therapists. From my personal experience as a patient and as a physician, it speaks the truth."
—Bernie Siegel, author of *Prescriptions for Living*

"...a welcome resource for individuals living with cancer and for all caregivers."
—Dawn Nelson, author of *From the Heart Through the Hands*

—*"...a unique comprehensive guide to the use of massage in helping cancer patients to heal. I highly recommend it for practitioners, patients and caregivers alike."*
—Joe Coletto, National College of Naturopathic Medicine

Medicine Hands debunks a pervasive health myth that massage is anathema for those suffering with cancer. The idea that cancer can metastasize as a result of massage is not rooted in any science. Touch and massage are vital to a cancer patient's health and well-being.

Medicine Hands is a practical book written for both health professionals and the lay person. Research is highlighted with anecdotes, stories, and vignettes of cancer patients, massage therapists, caregivers, hospice workers and other health professionals. Practical information is presented on administering touch, drug-related considerations, providing care at home, and dealing with hospital and hospice situations.

Medicine Hands is an invaluable resource for:
• Massage therapists and other touch therapists (e.g. Therapeutic Touch and Reiki)
• Cancer patients and their caregivers and families
• Oncologits and cancer treatment centers
• Natural health clinics
• Massage and other alternative medicine schools and educational settings
• Health care professionals — nurses, doctors, hospice workers — who come into contact with cancer patients

Gayle MacDonald, a long time health educator and veteran massage therapist, finds that her personal and professional interests are inseperable. It was after suffering ill health herself that she became the health and physical educator she had always wanted to be. She continues to teach in her native Oregon, helping others to expand their awareness that in massage they are performing a service that integrates the sacred with the mundane, and they not only touch their patients body, but also their heart, mind and soul.

PUBLISHED BY FINDHORN PRESS — SAME FORMAT AND SIZE AS FROM THE HEART THROUGH THE HANDS
ISBN 1-899171-77-0

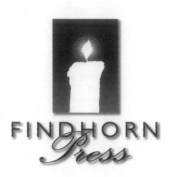

FINDHORN
Press

Findhorn Press is the publishing business of the Findhorn Community which has grown around the Findhorn Foundation in northern Scotland.

For further information about the Findhorn Foundation and the Findhorn Community, please contact:

Findhorn Foundation

The Visitors Centre
The Park, Findhorn IV36 3TY, Scotland, UK
tel 01309 690311• fax 01309 691301
email vcentre@findhorn.org
www.findhorn.org

For a complete Findhorn Press catalogue, please contact:

Findhorn Press

The Press Building, The Park,
Forres IV36 3TY
Scotland, UK
Tel 01309 690582
freephone 0800-389-9395
Fax 01309 690036
e-mail info@findhornpress.com
www.findhornpress.com

If you live in the USA or Canada, please send your request to:

Findhorn Press

c/o Lantern Books
1 Union Square West
New York, NY 10003